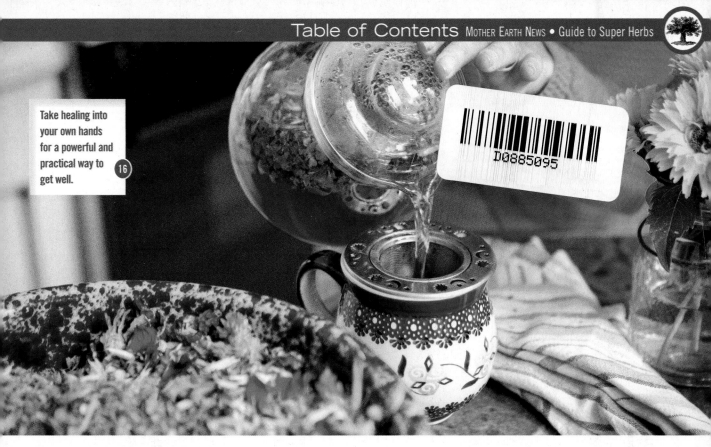

Take healing into your own hands for a powerful and practical way to get well. **16**

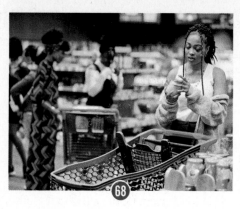
68

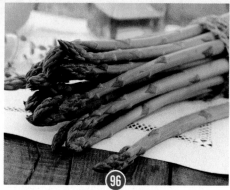
96

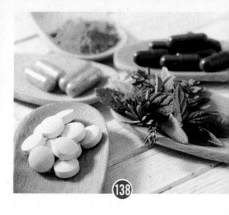
138

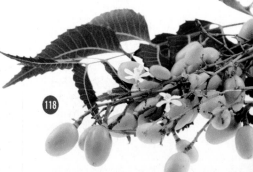
118

FIND MOTHER EARTH NEWS ONLINE

Visit MotherEarthNews.com to find more sustainable lifestyle articles, podcasts, and videos to help you on your journey to self-sufficient living, and be sure to subscribe to our weekly newsletters.

Herbal Respiratory Relief

If you suffer from chronic respiratory issues such as asthma or allergies, take comfort in some wonderful lung tonic herbs. Find remedies at MotherEarthNews.com/Herbal-Respiratory-Relief.

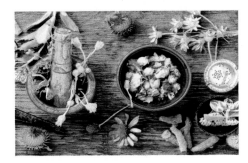

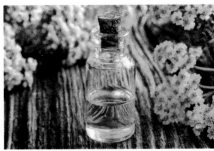

Distilling Hydrosol and Essential Oils

Join us as we demonstrate how to distill hydrosols, and provide tips on the extraction processes for both hydrosols and essential oils. Watch at home by visiting MotherEarthNews.com/Distilling-Hydrosols-Video.

Beginning Your Medicinal Herb Garden

Looking to start your very own medicinal garden? One long-time reader shares which herbs she recommends to someone just starting out so they don't feel overwhelmed. Find the article at MotherEarthNews.com/Beginning-Medicinal-Garden.

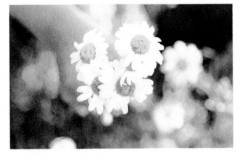

Heirlooms and Herbals Talk Yarrow

Kansas herbalist Joanne Bauman hosts MOTHER EARTH NEWS' natural health podcast, Heirlooms and Herbals. This episode explores the health and history of yarrow. Listen at home or on the go by visiting MotherEarthNews.com/Heirloom-Herbals-Yarrow.

Cleopatra's Aloe Vera Cleanser

Cleopatra's skin-care methods have stood the test of time. Cleanse, moisturize, and beautify your skin with a recipe inspired by this reigning beauty. Follow along at MotherEarthNews.com/Cleopatra-Aloe-Vera-Cleanser.

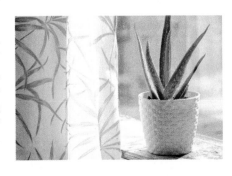

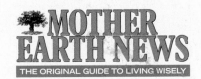

THE ORIGINAL GUIDE TO LIVING WISELY

COLLECTOR'S EDITION
GUIDE TO SUPER HERBS
WINTER 2020

Special Content Team
Issue Editor GINA DEBACKER
Group Editor JEAN TELLER

Convergent Media
BRENDA ESCALANTE
785-274-4404; bescalante@ogdenpubs.com

Art Direction and Pre-Press
Art Director AMANDA BARNWELL

Web and Digital Content
Digital Content Manager TONYA OLSON

Display Advertising
800-678-5779; adinfo@ogdenpubs.com

Newsstand
Newsstand Manager MELISSA GEIKEN

Customer Service
800-234-3368;
customerservice@ogdenpubs.com

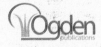

Publisher BILL UHLER
Circulation & Marketing Director CHERILYN OLMSTED
Newsstand & Production Director BOB CUCCINIELLO
Sales Director BOB LEGAULT
Director of Events & Business Development ANDREW PERKINS
Information Technology Director TIM SWIETEK
Finance & Accounting Director ROSS HAMMOND

MOTHER EARTH NEWS (ISSN 0027-1535)
is published bimonthly by Ogden Publications Inc.,
1503 SW 42nd St., Topeka, KS 66609.
For subscription inquiries call 800-234-3368.
Outside the U.S. and Canada, call 785-274-4365;
fax 785-274-4305.

© 2020 Ogden Publications Inc. Printed in the U.S.A.

1% FOR THE PLANET MEDIA · BBB · Certified B Corporation · Please Recycle This Magazine

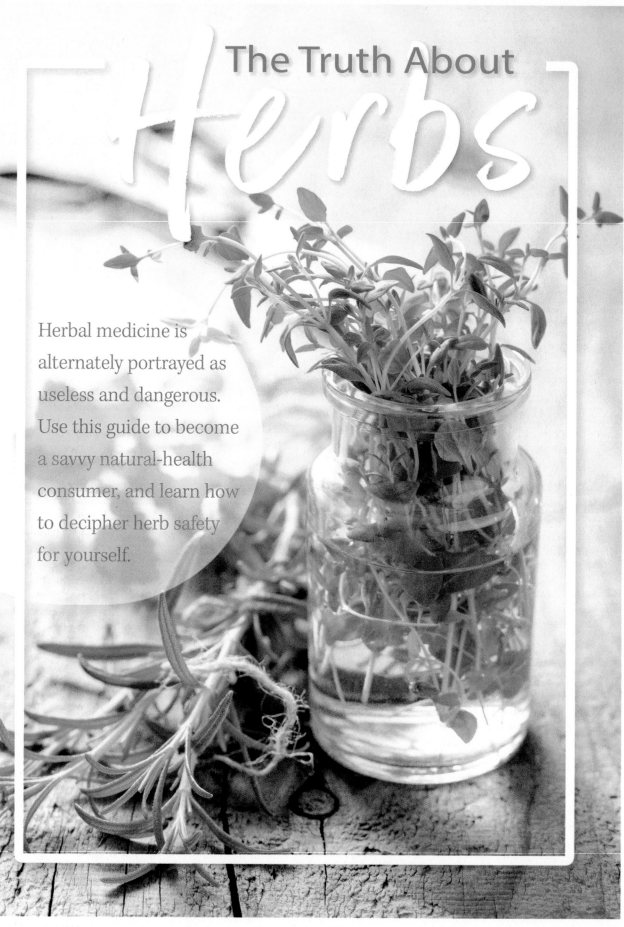

The Truth About Herbs

Herbal medicine is alternately portrayed as useless and dangerous. Use this guide to become a savvy natural-health consumer, and learn how to decipher herb safety for yourself.

Breaking News:

Is chamomile deadly? Why a recent study has experts wondering whether that cup of tea in your hand might just be a death sentence. Follow-up at 10 o'clock.

By Dawn Combs

These days, I watch the news looking for scare tactics like this. It can sometimes seem as if the media is actively trying to discredit herbal medicine. Because the average consumer doesn't know the full story behind each study, and often doesn't have the time, inclination, or tools to analyze the information themselves, they ditch the herbal option thinking, "better safe than sorry"—even though they may be skeptical that chamomile is dangerous. This is unfortunate when we consider the boon to wellness herbal medicines can be, especially when our mainstream medical system focuses more on treating symptoms than on promoting health.

The Herbal Environment

We herbal health advocates are in a sticky place in the U.S. The mainstream medical community often says herbal and botanical medicines are ineffective, while simultaneously saying herbal medicines are dangerous. The idea that the mainstream media may have motivation to discredit nonconventional medicine is one backed by research. As Mark Blumenthal, executive director of the American Botanical Council, stated in his 2013 speech, "Health Benefits of Popular Herbal Supplements in the U.S. Market" (find a link to speech at MotherEarthNews.com/Truth-About-Herbs), "If you look at medical journals, they too are subject to bias. According to a pilot trial of 11 top journals, the more advertising in a medical journal over a one-year period from pharmaceutical drug advertising, the less coverage there was on herbs and dietary supplements in general—and what coverage there was tended to be negative about safety and efficacy."

Along with creating a confusing environment for the average consumer, this also makes legislation governing the sale of herbal products a bit schizophrenic. It makes it possible for sketchy, and often dangerous, "natural" diet supplements to be sold by everyone from TV personalities to the corner drugstore. Then, when these supplements—which promise to help someone lose 50 pounds in two weeks with no effort—inevitably harm people, it casts doubt on natural products as a whole.

At Mockingbird Meadows Herbal Health Farm (MockingbirdMeadows.com), where we teach people how to grow, prepare, and use medicinal herbal applications, we advise our students to make the purest product they can in the cleanest manner possible. We suggest they comply with the laws and maintain superior customer service. This doesn't guarantee there will never be questions, but it can help assure the growing group of consumers who are seeking these products that the intent behind their creation is one of health.

Personal Wellness

Our current health-care system is unsustainable. Rather than focusing on common-sense, time-honored ways to improve our health and wellness, we live in unhealthful ways and then expect pharmaceutical medicine to undo the damage we've done to our bodies.

It's inappropriate to expect Western medicine to do more than the heroic, life-saving medicine it's very talented at performing. To maintain health, we can turn back to simple methods. As we take the load of daily wellness off our health-care system, we will increasingly turn to nature—meaning high-quality foods and well-researched herbal medicine, along with healthful habits such as exercising daily and reducing stress. That means we'll need to know how to demand and discern quality in our foods and herbs.

The three main areas that follow are where we consumers need to equip ourselves with good tools of discernment.

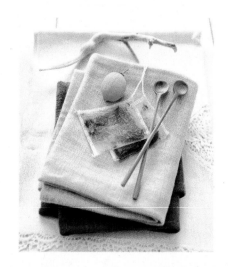

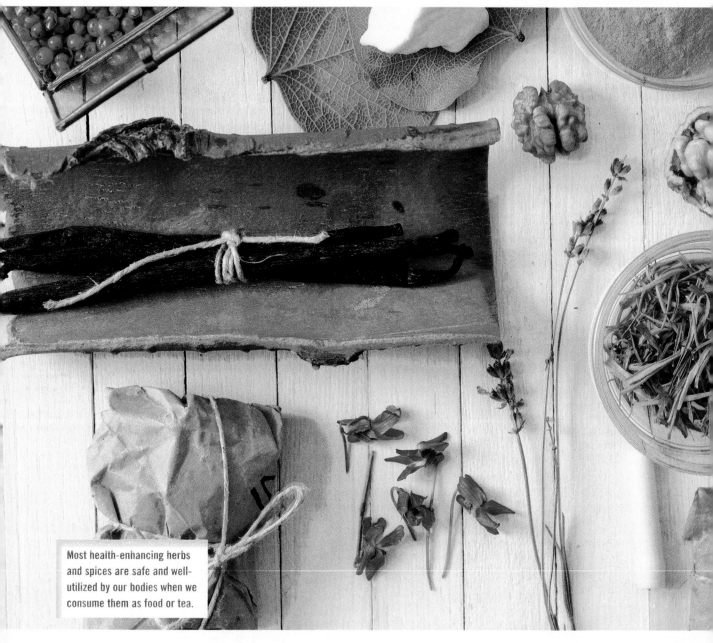

Most health-enhancing herbs and spices are safe and well-utilized by our bodies when we consume them as food or tea.

New Medical Studies

Although studies designed to test safety and confirm effectiveness of herbal medicines are abundant, they are frequently underreported or reported irresponsibly. This means we must educate ourselves beyond the headlines.

It can be difficult to find reliable reporting on herbal science, but the good news is that the studies are happening. "People say there's not enough science about herbs; I've heard some physicians say there's no science about herbs," Blumenthal says. "If you look at the data in the last 30 years, the number of studies on herbal preparation and isolated compounds have gone from 739 papers in 1977 to over 6,000 in 2007."

Comfrey (*Symphytum* spp.) makes a good case study. Some years ago, a study cast doubt on herbs that contain pyrrolizidine alkaloids (PAs)—in particular comfrey. As a result, comfrey is not on the FDA's generally recognized as safe (GRAS) list. The herbal community self-regulates by this list, agreeing to refrain from selling products containing comfrey that are intended for internal consumption. This is why you won't see it in a cough syrup in the store.

I use comfrey in many of my classes as an illustration of how to break down a study and make personal health-care decisions. When confronted with a breaking news bulletin about a study, it's important to ask the following:

- Who funded the research and what was their motivation?
- What are the methods of the research?
- What are the applications to human use?
- Was this trial on humans or animals?
- What is the historical information on the herb? Have there ever been any written indications of the same issue?
- What are your own personal decisions after reading the research, and what are the individual health concerns that must be factored into your decision?

Using these standards, let's look at comfrey more closely. Comfrey is the common name for a group of nine species of perennial plants in the genus *Symphytum*. Some of these species, including *S. officinale*, are known to contain pyrrolizidine alkaloids. Some members of the genus contain very small amounts or none at all, for example *S. ×uplandicum*, believed to be the native species in the U.S. Humans have a long-

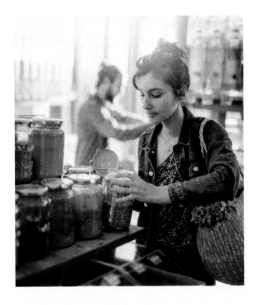

Buying Herbs & Herbal Products Safely

When it comes to herbal health-care products, it can be tough to learn much from labels. We recommend first researching responsible companies. Then, look for these indications of quality on product labels. All herbs listed should be designated by both their common name and their botanical name like this: Nettle (*Urtica dioica*). If the package doesn't identify the botanical name, this is cause for suspicion. A given herb may go by upwards of 100 common names, but there is only one botanical name—be certain you are getting the herb you intend.

The packaging should contain all necessary labeling: Herbal products should have the ingredients, instructions on use, the appropriate FDA warning verbiage, and contraindications. Although some manufacturers may not agree with the principles behind the need for "warnings," the intent of a person who doesn't take their product seriously enough to follow the law must factor into your decision to buy. (Consider the difference between buying something homegrown and something from a store shelf. Labeling on this level is perhaps not as important when someone is not running a business.)

Beware larger-than-life claims. Claims that the herb is a "cure" should set off warning alarms. Herbs should be considered partners in our bid for balanced health. They do important work in a body that is making changes in diet and lifestyle. No reputable product will claim to do all the work for you in a pill, tincture, tea, or cream.

written history of using plants from this genus for medicine without a cause for concern.

The study that started the controversy was done on 21-week-old rats, which don't have the same reaction to PAs as humans do. The rats were injected with a high dose of one of the isolated PAs (symphytine) rather than a dilution of the whole plant. When you isolate a compound within a plant, you do not get the thousands of other chemicals that often act as a buffer for that compound. At any rate, we don't inject comfrey, we eat it. When it is injected, the effect of the compound is concentrated. A small number of the rats in the study subsequently developed liver cancer. Were we to duplicate the same level of PA consumption used in the study in our daily diet, we would need to consume between three-quarters of a pound and 114 pounds a day for at least 21 weeks. Given that the average amount in a therapeutic dose is less than a quarter of an ounce, this is possible but highly unreasonable.

"The comfrey incident might have looked different if it had been put into context of a toxicity scale," Blumenthal says. "One such scale is the HERP (human exposure/rodent potency) index, which classifies the cancer-causing potentials of various substances. Extrapolating from the HERP index, former U.S. Department of Agriculture botanist James Duke calculates that less than one-fifth of an ounce of brown mustard is twice as cancer-causing as comfrey tea, which has roughly the same cancer-causing potential as a peanut butter sandwich. Wine is 144 times more cancer-causing than an equal amount of comfrey tea."

Finally, there is no information in the historic data of problems with the use of comfrey and there are no cases of veno-occlusive liver disease that can be definitively traced to its ingestion.

Many people continue to use comfrey internally without concern. In the U.S., if you are wild-harvesting or growing your own, you are very likely getting *S. ×uplandica* anyway—which doesn't contain the potentially concerning PAs. In all such cases, you must balance the newer scientific findings on each herb with your own internal voice. You may see no logical reason to avoid eating comfrey, but a family history of liver dysfunction makes you think twice. You may be ready to use it in your tea but have a niggling doubt in your gut. If so, comfrey isn't right for you. You can use comfrey externally without concern and avoid the internal controversy altogether. In the end, many other herbs may work as well or better for your particular body chemistry.

We must all be the arbiters of our own health. Regardless of any study or other people's experiences, not every herb is right for every person. Our bodies are all unique and therefore the ailments that befall us require specialized treatment.

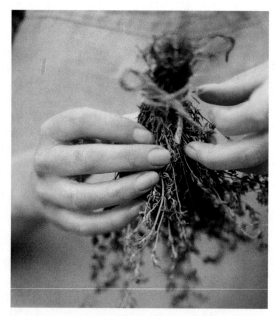

If a tried-and-true herb isn't benefitting your health, turn to another one. It might work better for your body.

Anytime you decide a "banned" herb is right for you, be sure to let your health-care team know of your decision so they can offer you their perspectives and help you avoid any future negative interactions or overuse.

Personal Medicine

We must all be the arbiters of our own health. Regardless of any study or other people's experiences, not every herb is right for every person. Our bodies are all unique and therefore the ailments that befall us require specialized treatment.

Valerian may be the perfect herb for you to combat your insomnia. Unfortunately, my husband is one of a small percentage of people for whom valerian is a stimulant. Instead of sleeping, when I once gave him valerian tincture before bed, he stayed up most of the night organizing my kitchen cupboards. Nice for me; bad for him.

For nearly any health ailment, there are specific herbs practitioners find to be successful again and again throughout the history of their use. There is also a long list of other herbs that might work just as well. If you try an herb that everyone suggests as "specific" for your problem and it fails, don't be discouraged. Instead, try a different herb. My husband did very well with hops instead of valerian.

Adulteration

Finally, when it comes to herbal preparations, quality is of utmost importance. Adulteration can mean that the herb in question is being mixed with something else at the point of processing. It's fairly common in unscrupulous facilities to "cut" the more expensive herb with a more common plant as filler. Profits go up, and sadly sometimes so do the incidences of toxicity. In many cases, we are able to analyze the herb and its constituents and show that none of the chemicals found normally in the plant can cause the damage in question.

Kava (*Piper methysticum*) is a recent example of this problem. A decade ago, concerns surfaced over the possible hepatotoxicity of the herb, which is traditionally used to treat anxiety and insomnia. In the case against kava, it was believed that there were 50 to 100 possible incidences of toxicity from the plant. This equates to a chance of liver damage possibility to one in every 1 million daily doses. That's a pretty low chance of liver damage, especially from an herb that has been used without incident for hundreds of years. Nonetheless, it warranted that the herbal community pause and look at the data we had. The German Commission E put a stop to anyone marketing kava products in Europe, and here in the U.S., kava disappeared from the shelves.

But why was kava, which has been used for many years without incident, suddenly causing toxicity problems? One of the best theories is that instead of using only the root, as has been done throughout the history of using this plant, the leaves and stems were added. The substance pipermethystine is present in the aboveground parts of the plant and not in the root. It also happens to be hepatotoxic. Another possibility is that in the process of creating tinctures of kava, some manufacturers may have inadvertently introduced toxic substances as part of their tincturing process.

Recently, a German court lifted the effectual ban on kava. The risk-to-benefit ratio favors the benefits of this plant—the medicine used to replace its effects has more risk. Controversy will most likely continue to swirl around kava.

Regardless of the herbs you choose for yourself or your family, it's important to keep in mind the stipulations at right. 🌿

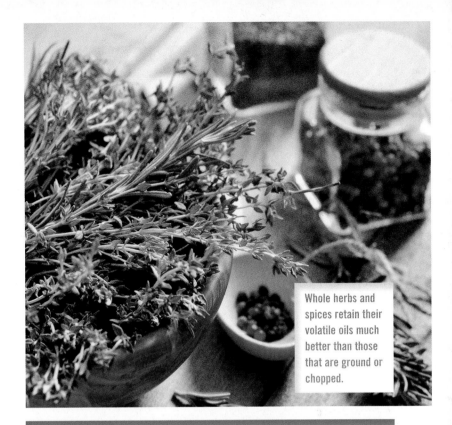

Whole herbs and spices retain their volatile oils much better than those that are ground or chopped.

- Buy only from reputable sources. Choose established herbal wholesalers whose business practices demonstrate their intention to source responsibly.
- Make your own tinctures.
- Use the herb in the way it was intended. When used occasionally for short periods of anxiety and stress, kava shines. It has not traditionally been taken every day in a therapeutic dose.
- Memberships to organizations such as the American Botanical Council can provide you with access to peer-reviewed studies on herbs used for medicinal purposes.

Dawn Combs is the owner of Mockingbird Meadows Herbal Health Farm in central Ohio and the director of its Eclectic Herbal Institute (MockingbirdMeadows. com). Combs is the author of *Sweet Remedies* and *Heal Local*, both of which are available at MotherEarthNews.com/Store.

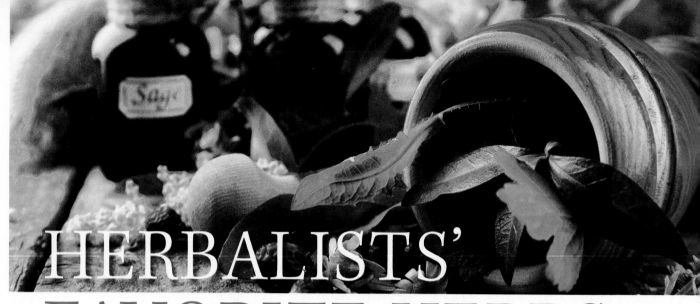

HERBALISTS' FAVORITE HERBS

Discover outstanding herbs for a range of health concerns
with these expert recommendations.

We asked some of our favorite herbalists to name their favorite medicinal herbs. The result is a list of five herbs that can come in handy in any medicine cabinet. In fact, many of these herbal stars can be taken on a long-term basis to support our overall health.

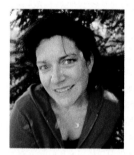

Dawn Combs

An ethnobotanist, educator, and *Mother Earth Living* contributor, Combs' experiences supporting her own health and that of her family have led to the practical education she provides online at HealLocal. com; in her classes at Mockingbird Meadows (MockingbirdMeadows. com); and through her nationally recognized product line of botanical supplements. She believes everyone can take charge of their health by reclaiming the knowledge of our ancestors, using modern medicine wisely and connecting with the natural world. She is the author of *Heal Local*, available at MotherEarthNews. com/Store.

ASHWAGNDHA FOR IMMUNITY: Ashwagndha (*Withania somnifera*) is my favorite herb for anyone who needs a stronger immune system. Common plants such as ginger and garlic are there for us when we're sick, but with an adaptogen like ashwagandha we can build our health and reduce the negative effects of stress to the point that we need intervention less.

■ **USAGE:** The root of this tropical plant from the tomato family (Solanaceae) can be decocted for a tea, tinctured, or used in capsule form by anyone who is not pregnant or hyperthyroid.

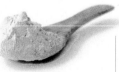

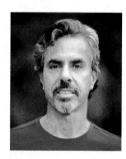

Chris Kilham

Medicine hunter Chris Kilham is a TV personality and author who has conducted medicinal plant research in more than 40 countries, helping popularize medicinal plants globally through media. He is the author of 15 books, including *The Ayahuasca Test Pilots Handbook* and the best-selling yoga book *The Five Tibetans*. Visit his website at MedicineHunter.com.

SCHISANDRA FOR MENTAL CLARITY: The beautiful berry of schisandra (*Schisandra chinensis*) boasts millennia of traditional uses for counteracting the aging process, for increasing energy, for fighting fatigue, and as a sexual tonic. It's considered one of the most highly protective of all medicinal plants. Schisandra offers special benefits for the mind. Several human studies show schisandra extract improves mental concentration, coordination, and endurance. Schisandra helps prevent mental fatigue and can increase accuracy and quality of work. In various human clinical studies with doctors, students, soldiers, and other groups, schisandra demonstrated superior mind-sharpening powers.

■ **USAGE:** Consider two capsules daily, or try a ¼ teaspoon of concentrated schisandra powder in water or juice.

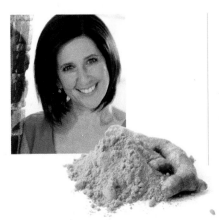

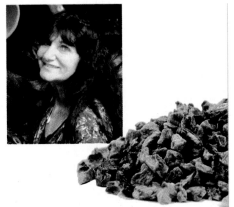

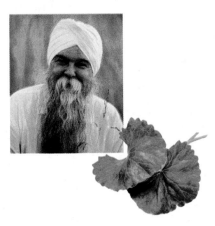

Aviva Romm

For more than three decades, Aviva Romm has bridged traditional medicine with good science. A midwife, herbalist, and Yale-trained M.D., Romm is also Board Certified in Family Medicine with Obstetrics, as well as a graduate of Dr. Andrew Weil's Integrative Medicine Residency through the University of Arizona. Her focus is on women's and children's health, with an emphasis on the impact of stress on health, food cravings, weight, chronic disease, and hormone imbalance. Romm is one of the nation's leaders in the field of botanical medicine and is the author of seven books, including the textbook *Botanical Medicine for Women's Health*.

TURMERIC FOR ARTHRITIS: Curcumin—an active anti-inflammatory constituent in the traditional food seasoning turmeric (*Curcuma longa*)—is almost always included in my prescriptions to my patients struggling with arthritis (both osteoarthritis and rheumatoid arthritis). The anti-inflammatory effects, as well as support for systemic detoxification in those with rheumatoid arthritis, are an important part of treatment.

■ **USAGE:** I typically recommend 1,000 mg one to two times a day. It's safe for most people to take daily and for an extended time. I love to combine it with ginger, an anti-inflammatory that has been shown to be as effective as NSAIDs such as aspirin and ibuprofen for pain—a factor in both types of arthritis. For ginger, I suggest 250 to 500 mg one to two times daily in capsules.

Rosemary Gladstar

A star figure in the field of modern herbalism, Rosemary Gladstar is internationally renowned for her technical knowledge and stewardship in the herbalist community. She has been learning, teaching, and writing about herbs for more than 40 years and is the author of 11 books. Gladstar co-founded Traditional Medicinals Wellness Teas; founded The California School of Herbal Studies; is the Founding President of United Plant Savers; and is the director of the International Herb Symposium and The New England Women's Herbal Conference. She lives and works from Sage Mountain Herbal Retreat Center and Botanical Sanctuary. Visit her website at SageMountain.com.

RHODIOLA FOR STRESS: If I had to choose one herb for long-term stress, it would the fabulous adaptogen rhodiola (*Rhodiola rosea*). This beautiful little succulent helps us adapt to the stresses of our full and busy lives. Not an evening tea, rhodiola is better in the morning as it provides energy for the day.

■ **USAGE:** To take as a tea, blend 1 part rhodiola with ½ part cinnamon and ½ part ginger. Use 1 to 2 teaspoons of the mix per cup, simmering lightly for 15 minutes. Drink 1 to 2 cups in the morning. To take rhodiola in tincture form, put ½ teaspoon tincture in ¼ cup warm water with a bit of lemon or lime. **Note:** Wild rhodiola grown in remote areas such as Siberia has been overharvested. I'm delighted to see more U.S.-grown organic rhodiola sources available now.

K.P. Khalsa

Karta Purkh Singh Khalsa, a nationally registered herbalist and certified Ayurvedic practitioner, has been practicing herbalism for 45 years. Khalsa is a state-credentialed dietitian-nutritionist, president emeritus of the American Herbalists Guild, director for the National Ayurvedic Medical Association, and a teacher at Bastyr University and National College of Natural Medicine.

GOTU KOLA FOR VITALITY: This unassuming member of the parsley family, often called brahmi, is a treasure chest of benefits for tissue healing and mental functioning. Used as food (in salads, sauces, and drinks) and as medicine in high-dose tea, gotu kola (*Centella asiatica*) is recommended in all three of the world's major traditional herbal systems. It fortifies nerve tissue and memory, and heals skin and joints.

■ **USAGE:** For acute use, such as in the case of clinically diagnosed cognitive decline, nerve injury, or a connective tissue condition, brew 60 grams gotu kola as tea. Enjoy a beverage-strength cup of tea daily for long-term health. ❧

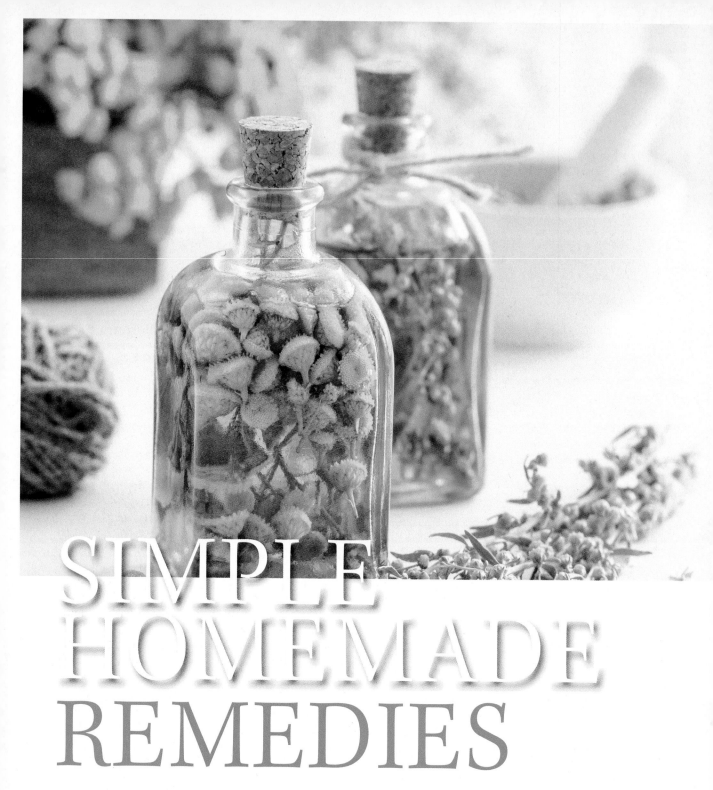

SIMPLE HOMEMADE REMEDIES

Make your own simple,
effective herbal remedies,
and add medicine-
making to your self-
sufficiency repertoire.

By Michelle Schoffro Cook

Making our own herbal medicines and body-care products can save money and improve our health, and it's much easier than you may think. If you already make herbal teas, then making infusions, decoctions, tinctures, salves, and poultices can quickly become part of your repertoire, too. Don't worry if they sound confusing; you'll soon discover how to prepare a variety of plants to make a range of simple but effective herbal medicines.

One very important note before you begin making herbal medicines: Always make sure you are using the correct plant (check the Latin name) and the correct part of the plant (flower, leaf, roots), as some parts may be toxic if used internally.

Internal Medicines

Making herbal tea may seem fairly straightforward, but to reap the greatest medicinal value from herbs, we need to do more than dunk a tea bag in hot water. There are two main forms of herbal tea: infusions and decoctions.

■ **Infusions:** Infusions are the commonly known form of herbal tea, in which herbs are literally infused in hot water, usually 1 heaping teaspoon of dried herb (or one tea bag) per cup of hot water for 10 to 20 minutes. This is the ideal method for extracting the medicinal compounds in most berries, flowers, and leaves. You can also use fresh herbs, but because of their higher water content, you usually need to double the amount of herbal matter per cup of water (2 teaspoons per cup of water instead of one).

■ **Decoctions:** To extract the medicinal compounds from seeds, roots, or stems, you'll want to make a decoction, which involves boiling the herbs and allowing them to simmer for about an hour, usually allowing 1 heaping teaspoon of dried herb per cup of water. Note that this method is less suitable for berries, flowers, and leaves because it tends to destroy many of the delicate medicinal compounds they contain. As with infusions, you can use fresh herbs, but you typically need to double the amount of herb matter per cup of water.

What if you want to make a tea from some combination of roots, berries, seeds, stems, flowers, and leaves? Start by making a decoction with the roots, seeds, or stems. Bring it to a boil, then reduce to a simmer to continue brewing for an hour. Turn off the heat and add any berries, flowers, or leaves. Allow the mixture to steep for an additional 10 to 20 minutes. Now you've extracted the best medicinal compounds from all of the herbal components you're using.

■ **Tinctures:** Tinctures are alcohol extracts of fresh or dried herbs. They're highly effective at preserving a plant's active constituents. You can make a tincture from roots, leaves, seeds, stems, or even its flowers.

To make an herbal tincture, finely chop the fresh, clean herb you are using. You can also use dried herbs. Either way, the idea is to chop the herb as much as possible to give the alcohol as much surface area to act upon as you can. Some herbalists recommend grinding dried herbs in a coffee/spice grinder before making a tincture.

Place the chopped or ground herb in a half-quart or quart-sized glass jar. Fill the jar with as much plant matter as possible to ensure the medicinal value of your tincture, keeping in mind that you'll need enough alcohol to completely submerge the herbal matter. Top with vodka or pure grain alcohol, making sure all of the plant matter is submerged in the alcohol to prevent mold growth. Note that different kinds of alcohol will produce different kinds of tinctures. Visit MountainRoseBlog.com/Guide-Tinctures-Extracts for more information. Date and label the jar, and allow the mixture to sit for two weeks, shaking daily to encourage extraction. After two weeks, strain the contents through a cheesecloth-lined sieve. After most of the liquid has gone through the sieve, pull up the corners of the cheesecloth and, using clean hands, carefully wring out any remaining liquid.

Store the herbal tincture in a dark glass jar or dropper bottle away from heat or sunlight to preserve its healing properties. Tinctures will usually keep for a few years. You can make an herbal tincture out of any medicinal or culinary herb that can be used internally. A typical tincture dose is 30 drops (about one dropperful) three times daily, but we recommend looking up specific dosage recommendations for the herbs you use. Avoid tinctures if you are pregnant or nursing, or if you have liver disease, diabetes, or alcoholism.

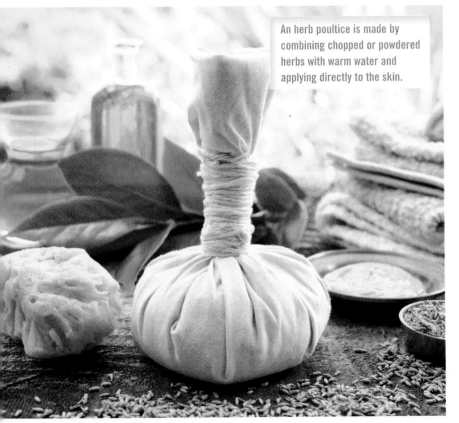

An herb poultice is made by combining chopped or powdered herbs with warm water and applying directly to the skin.

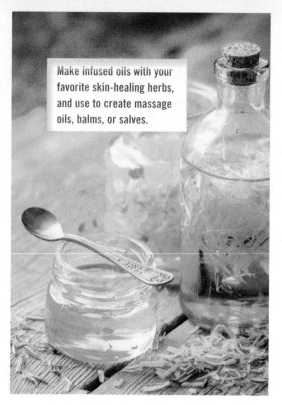

Make infused oils with your favorite skin-healing herbs, and use to create massage oils, balms, or salves.

Some of My Favorite Healing Herbs

All of the herbs listed here are safe and effective. However, before making specific remedies on your own, research the herb you plan to use to ensure you're using the right parts and amounts, as well as contraindications that may apply specifically to you and your circumstances.

CALENDULA (FLOWERS): Skin healer extraordinaire

CHAMOMILE (FLOWERS): Relaxant and dental antimicrobial (use tea as a mouthwash)

DANDELION (ROOTS OR LEAVES): Osteoporosis preventer and anticancer powerhouse

ECHINACEA (ROOTS): Immune booster

FEVERFEW (FLOWERS AND LEAVES): Headache and migraine alleviator

GARLIC (CLOVES): Amazing germ buster

GINGER (ROOT): Muscle and joint pain healer

HORSETAIL (LEAVES): Nail, teeth, and bone builder

JUNIPER (BERRIES): Urinary tract antimicrobial

LAVENDER (FLOWERS): Anxiety and depression alleviator

LICORICE (ROOT): Chronic fatigue syndrome solution

NETTLES (LEAVES): Allergy remedy

OREGANO (LEAVES): Antimicrobial antidote

PEPPERMINT (LEAVES): Headache remedy and sinusitis aid

RED CLOVER (FLOWERS): Relieves menopausal symptoms such as hot flashes

ROSEMARY (LEAVES): Memory booster

ST. JOHN'S WORT (FLOWERS): Anxiety antidote and anticancer therapy; skin healer

THYME (LEAVES): Cough and anti-bacterial medicine

Sidebar adapted from Be Your Own Herbalist: Essential Herbs for Health, Beauty, and Cooking *by Michelle Schoffro Cook, PhD, DNM. To order, visit www.MotherEarthNews.com/Store.*

Skin-Healing Medicines

■ **Infused Oils:** Infused oils are made by infusing herbs in oil, rather than alcohol as in tinctures. The infusion technique works to transfer the healing properties of herbs to oils. Infused oils are excellent for massage; as skin or bath oils; or as a basis for balms and salves, which I'll explain in the next section. Never ingest these oils.

Infused oils are easy to make. Choose any type of vegetable or carrier oil, other than petrochemical-based oils such as baby oil or mineral oil. It's also best to avoid oils that break down quickly when exposed to heat such as flax seed oil. I prefer olive oil or sweet almond oil, which can be warmed to encourage the transfer of healing compounds from the herb matter to the oil.

You can make many types of infused oils, but two of the most common are St. John's wort and calendula oils. St. John's wort oil, made from the flowers of the plant, can be used for treating bruises, swellings, hemorrhoids, scars, and sprains. It's also recommended as a topical treatment for eczema. Avoid sun exposure for a few hours after using this oil on your skin as it can cause photosensitivity. Calendula oil, also made from the flowers of the plant, aids wound healing and alleviates various skin conditions.

Making herbal infused oils is particularly suited for the delicate flowers and leaves of a plant. Simply add fresh flowers or leaves

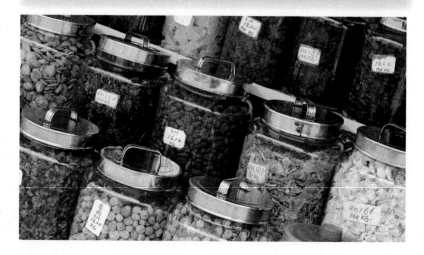

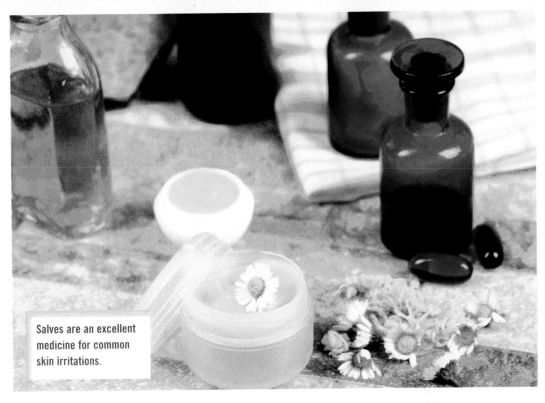

to a jar and fill it with oil such as sweet almond oil, apricot kernel oil, almond oil, or olive oil. You'll want enough plant matter to ensure the medicinal value of the infused oil, but not packed so tightly that the oil cannot penetrate the plant material. The plant material must be completely submerged in the oil to prevent mold from forming. Label and date the jar, including the herb and the oil used. Allow the infusion to rest for two weeks, shaking the bottle periodically to encourage the infusion process. After two weeks, strain the herbs from the oil, squeezing out any remaining oil with clean hands. Cap and label the jar, and store away from light and heat.

Salves are an excellent medicine for common skin irritations.

■ **Salves:** Salves are herbal balms or ointments made by thickening herbal oil infusions with melted beeswax. Most health-food stores sell plain beeswax, which can be shaved with a potato peeler or grated with a cheese grater and then melted over low heat. You can also buy beeswax pastilles, which are ready to melt. Be sure to avoid other types of wax as they are made of petroleum byproducts.

Allow 2 tablespoons of shaved, melted beeswax to 1 cup of infused oil after the herbal material has been strained off. Melt the oil and beeswax over low heat, preferably in a double-boiler, to prevent overheating. Be sure to stir regularly. Remove from the heat as soon as the beeswax is melted and well-incorporated into the oil. Immediately pour into small, shallow jars, tins, or lip balm containers. Let cool undisturbed to allow the ointment to set. Use for skin irritations and other skin conditions, and for dry or chapped lips. Similar to herbal infusions, calendula and St. John's wort are excellent choices to use in salves.

■ **Poultices:** A poultice is a paste made with herbs that is applied to the skin. It's typically applied while hot or warm, except when made with herbs that are naturally chemically hot such as chilies or ginger. To make a poultice, fill a natural-fiber cloth bag with powdered or chopped fresh herb matter. Tie it closed, and then place it in a bowl of hot water just long enough to soak and heat the herb. Remove it from the water, and apply to the affected area until the poultice has cooled and until you experience some relief. Reheat and reapply the poultice. It's best to use a fresh poultice each day.

Poultices are very effective in soothing aching or painful joints or muscles, as is the case with ginger. Calendula helps bruises and damaged skin, while echinacea boosts the immune system to help heal long-lasting wounds. 🌿

Michelle Schoffro Cook is the author of *Be Your Own Herbalist*, *60 Seconds to Slim*, and *The Probiotic Promise*; all are available atMotherEarthNews.com/ Store. Visit DrMichelleCook.com and WorldsHealthiestDiet.com to learn more about her work.

Basic Skin-Healing Salve
Ingredients
- 3 ounces calendula- and chamomile- infused oil
- ½ ounce pure beeswax
- 15 drops lavender essential oil
- Three 1-ounce salve jars

Directions: Slowly heat infused oil in a saucepan to about 100 degrees. Chop or grate the beeswax and gradually stir it into hot oil. Once beeswax is melted, remove from heat and stir in essential oil.

Pour hot salve into 1-ounce jars and let cool. Cap jars after it has cooled and store at room temperature.

Michelle Schoffro Cook

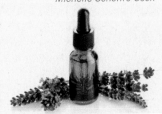

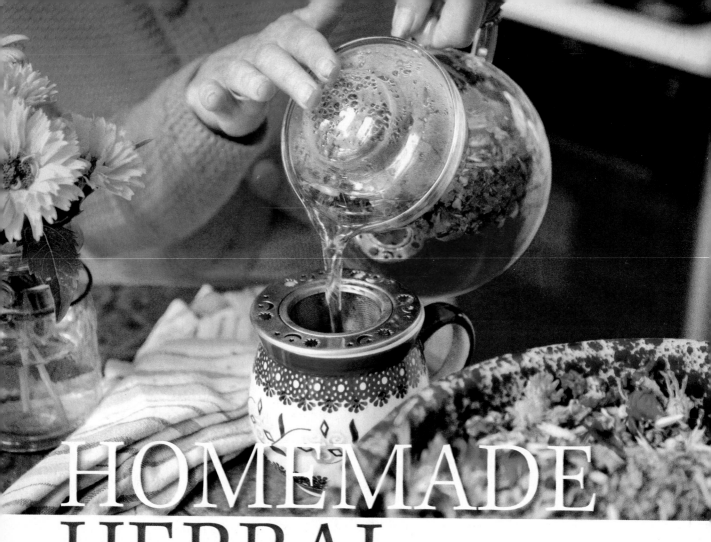

HOMEMADE HERBAL MEDICINES

Simple and safe, these powerhouse plant remedies
can help you heal on a shoestring.

By Stephen Harrod Buhner

Somewhat glumly, I celebrated my 61st birthday this past July. In the back of my mind, I've been sure for 45 years that God would make an exception to my normal and natural biodegrading process, thus allowing me to remain 35 years old well into my 90s. Somehow, it escaped the Universe's notice that some fine print in my birth contract negates, in my case, the aging process. A failing I am trying to get across, without success (so far).

In general, however, I am very healthy and I do have one very special thing going for me: I don't use any pharmaceuticals, unlike nearly everyone I know in my age group. On the rare occasion I do visit a physician, that statement always generates a great deal of surprise. It is, as I have found, a very unusual event in these early decades of the 21st century. (It wasn't when I was young.)

The reason I don't take even one prescription pharmaceutical every day is mostly due to my lifestyle—primarily because of my reliance on herbal medicines. I have been using homemade herbal remedies as my primary health care for about 30 years. I've successfully treated everything from minor colds,

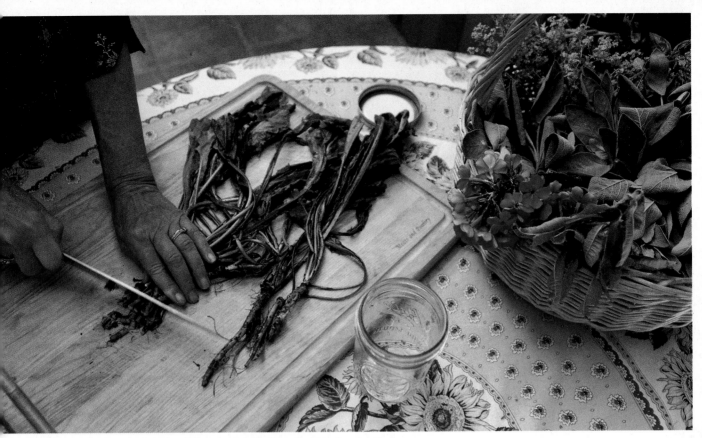

Take your healing into your own hands for a powerful and practical way to get well.

flus, cuts, and scrapes, which we all encounter on our journey through life, to irritable bowel syndrome and staph—with visits to many interesting conditions in between. Although herbal medicines may not be right for everyone's lifestyle, I have found the natural approach life-enhancing, self-empowering, inexpensive, and safe.

The best treatments I've found for common ailments all use herbs you can grow in your garden or likely have in your kitchen cupboards, disguised as condiments and spices. And, of course, these remedies are not the final answer on what works; nearly every plant you see around you can heal something.

Skin Conditions

Burns. I usually just pace around while verbally—and loudly—exploring the world of expletives. But sometimes I also use the following remedies.

1. Honey: This is especially good for severe burns. It will stop infection, stimulate skin regeneration, and keep the burned area moist. Honey is better for burns than nearly all medical interventions, even for third-degree burns.

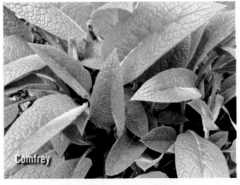
Comfrey

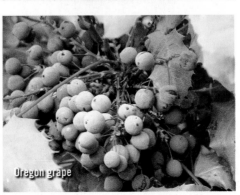
Oregon grape

Some plants' roots are medicinally potent. Comfrey root prompts healing, and Oregon grape root is a disinfectant.

2. Prickly pear cactus pads, filleted: Wear gloves to hold the pads while using a sharp knife to gently fillet the exterior skin off the pads. You will be left with slimy, oval pads of plant matter. Place the pads directly on the burn and bandage the wound. For a sunburn, rub the pads on the affected area.

Cuts and scrapes. Every one of us encounters life's sharp edges, often over and over again. Here's how I handle the aftereffects.

1. Wound powder: My homemade wound powder stops the bleeding, dries out the wound, inhibits infection, and stimulates healing. I generally use a bandage the first day and then leave the wound open afterward (unless it's in a hard-to-protect area or is gaping).

A good wound powder recipe contains any berberine plant (such as barberry, goldenseal, or Oregon grape root); comfrey root or leaf; juniper needles (the older the needles on the tree or bush, the better—old needles contain more tannins and will thus stop bleeding faster than young needles will); and maybe oregano, rosemary, or thyme. The berberine plant and juniper needles will disinfect, and

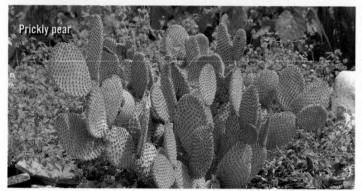
Bearberry

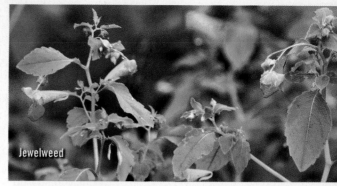
Jewelweed

Prickly pear

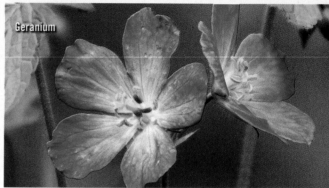
Geranium

Medicines derived from a variety of plant parts can heal many ailments, from burns to bacterial infections.

the juniper needles will also stop the bleeding. Comfrey will stimulate healing, and oregano, rosemary, and thyme are also antibacterials. I usually make the following recipe and keep it in the freezer to retain freshness:

Measure out 1 ounce of the berberine plant root or bark, ½ ounce of the comfrey root, 1 ounce of the juniper needles, and ¼ ounce of the oregano, rosemary, or thyme leaves (optional). Combine the ingredients, mix them in a blender or food processor until well-ground, and then powder the mixture until fine in a clean coffee grinder. I often sieve it afterward to get as flour-like a powder as possible. Sprinkle it liberally on the wound.

2. Honey: Stop using the wound powder after a few days and switch to honey. It's effective against all known drug-resistant bacteria and really speeds healing. Just cover the wound with honey, bandage, and change the dressing daily.

3. Wound salve: Use a combination of berberine plants, black walnut hulls, comfrey root, oregano leaves, rosemary leaves, Siberian elm bark (*Ulmus pumila*), and dried thyme. Add ¼ cup each of the roughly ground herbs to a baking dish and mix. Coat the blend with olive oil, cover the dish, and bake overnight in an oven on its lowest heat setting. In the morning, let the mixture cool. Press out and then reheat the oil. Stir in finely chopped or grated beeswax—2 ounces per cup of infused oil—and let melt. To check hardness, put a drop of salve on a plate and wait until the salve cools. It should remain solid but melt after a second of pressing on it with your finger.

Rashes. Rashes come in many forms, so treatments will vary. Here are a few.

1. For hives: Apply a tincture of *Echinacea angustifolia* root topically, using a cotton ball to administer it to the affected areas. Take ½ teaspoon of the tincture internally each hour

or so as well. (Pass on *E. purpurea*—I've found it useless for hives.)

2. For poison ivy: Jewelweed salve is best. Good additives are calendula flowers, chamomile flowers, and Siberian elm bark, all of which will soothe skin. Add any other herbs you want, but use the aerial parts of a jewelweed plant for half of the dried herbs by weight. Then, follow the same process as described earlier for making the wound salve.

Stings and bites. Use prickly pear as you would for burns or echinacea as you would for hives.

Intestinal Upsets

Diarrhea. Any strongly astringent plant will work for ordinary diarrhea. Blackberry root, the main standby used for millenia, is extremely effective. Krameria root, older pine needles just pulled off the tree, and wild geranium (*Geranium maculatum*) are all very helpful for regulation. To use, roughly chop or grind the dried herb of your choice. Add 1 ounce to a quart jar that can take heat, and fill with hot water. Cover the concoction and let it steep overnight (or for two hours if you really can't wait). Drink it throughout the next day. Repeat as needed.

Irritable bowel syndrome. Juice 1 beet, 1 piece of green cabbage (about the size of a medium carrot), 3 carrots, 4 stalks of celery and 4 leaves of fresh plantain (*Plantago* spp.). Plantain is a common plant you can usually find growing in front yards, and is unrelated to the banana of the same name. Cabbage and plantain are the most important ingredients, but they don't taste very good by themselves. The other ingredients will improve the taste while assisting your adrenal glands, liver, and immune system. Drink this juice every morning for breakfast, eat oatmeal for lunch, and have whatever you want for dinner. Irritable bowel syndrome will clear fairly rapidly on this regimen.

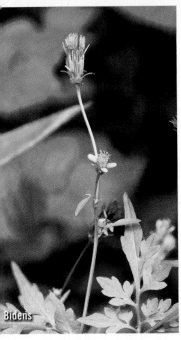
Bidens

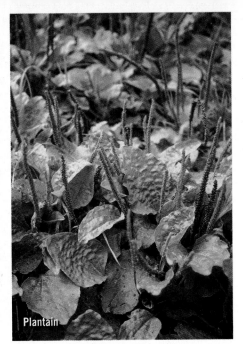
Plantain

Some common "weeds" with healing properties are likely growing right in your yard.

Viruses and Infections

Colds and flu. Many plants have antiviral properties—plants get colds just like we do, but because they can't go to the doctor, they make their own medicines. One of the best antiviral remedies is ginger, but use the fresh juice or it won't work. When cold and flu season approaches, I buy about a pound of fresh ginger and juice it. Make sure you squeeze out the pulp—a lot more juice will be in there. Put the ginger juice in any handy bottle and keep it the refrigerator. If everyone around me is getting sick or I feel that first onset of illness, I stir together 3 fluid ounces of the juice, 1 tablespoon of honey, a sprinkle of cayenne, the juice of a quarter of a lime, and 6 fluid ounces of hot water. Drink this blend as a hot tea three to six times per day. This tea rarely fails to either stop an infection's progression or heal it altogether. It's pretty good for opening up the sinuses as well.

Urinary tract infections. Juniper berries are highly effective for urinary tract infections. Bearberry (*Arctostaphylos uva-ursi*) is nearly as useful, and berberines are handy, too. I make a tincture of juniper berries—works like a charm. To make the tincture, take 1 ounce of dried juniper berries, grind them as finely as you can, and add 5 fluid ounces of a 50 percent alcoholic beverage such as vodka. Let the tincture steep for two weeks, decant it, press the berries to drain them of liquid, strain the tincture, and keep it in a bottle. Take 10 drops six times per day until the infection clears. If you use bearberry in place of juniper berries, take 30 drops six times daily. You can do the same if using a berberine plant.

Bidens also works for urinary tract infections. Bidens species constitute a fairly large grouping of plants, and all of the species you're likely to encounter are very good herbal medicines. They are sometimes called "beggar's ticks" (and even worse names), so you might be familiar with them under another moniker. Bidens plants are invasive and they grow pretty much everywhere. Bidens is a reliable, broad-spectrum antibacterial herb if you make a tincture from the fresh plant (dried bidens is useless for this). Pick bidens during or slightly before the plants are flowering. Cut up the plant, weigh it, and put 6 ounces in a jar. Add 12 fluid ounces of pure grain alcohol. You can use vodka, but the resulting medicine won't be as strong. Let the mixture steep for two weeks, decant it, strain and press the herbs to drain them well, and bottle the liquid. Use when needed.

Bidens is good for general systemic bacterial infections, but it's specifically useful for infections in mucus membrane systems. If you have a urinary tract infection and almost get well but then have a relapse, bidens is the perfect plant to use. Take ¼ to ½ teaspoon of the tincture up to six times per day for two to four weeks. Bidens is safe, and it hasn't failed me yet. *Bidens pilosa* is what most people use, but I use *B. pinnata* from my yard. Any bidens plant will most likely do.

Recommended Reading

To learn more about herbal medicines, I recommend *Making Plant Medicine* by Richo Cech, *The Herbal Medicine-Maker's Handbook* by James Green, and my book *Herbal Antibiotics*, second edition, which contains a *materia medica* of more than 200 plants and their medicinal preparation methods. These books explain in-depth how to make nearly all of the herbal medicines you'll ever need to use.

Wholesome Healing

The plant medicines that grow in our yards or sit in our kitchens can fairly easily heal most common ailments. I have found that after your life is saved by a plant, nothing is ever the same again. Herbal medicines open up a new world to the perceiving self. All of us who read Mother Earth News know we should work to help heal the earth, but your perspective will change significantly after you've experienced the earth healing you. ❦

Stephen Harrod Buhner is a renowned herbalist and the author of 19 books, including *Herbal Antibiotics* and *Herbal Antivirals* (order: MotherEarthNews.com/Store). He lives in Silver City, New Mexico.

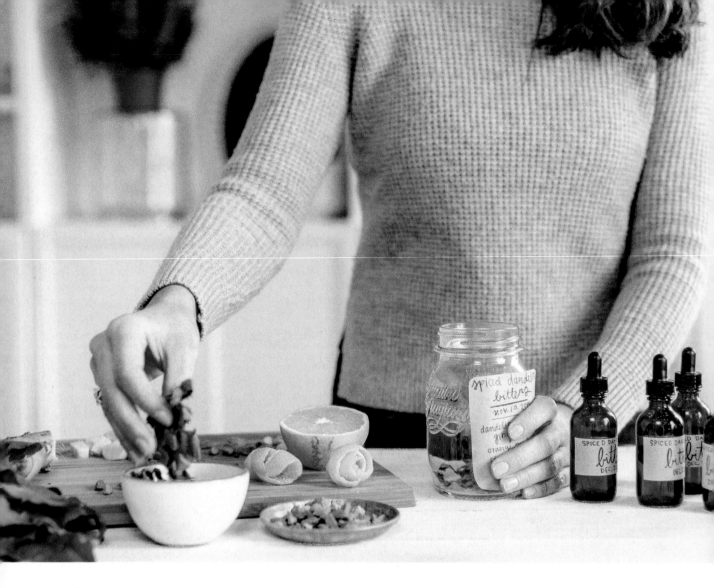

Winter's Best Herbal Remedies

Improve your health with bitters, elixirs, syrups, and vinegars — traditional herbal remedies perfect for winter.

By Gina DeBacker

Along with the beauty of snow-glistened trees and the festivity of holiday parties, winter also brings the onset of colds, flu, sore throats, and other ailments. Stocking our homes with time-tested, tried-and-true homemade remedies (and potent preventives) is a smart solution. These winter favorites come straight from Grandma's cupboard — from medicinal syrups and vinegars to sweet elixirs and old-fashioned bitters.

Note: Herbal medicines are used for their potential effects in the body; always discuss any new remedy with your doctor to make sure it's a good fit for you.

Always consult your health-care provider when considering treatments for children younger than 2.

Syrups

Some of the best herbal remedies for colds and sore throats are medicinal syrups. These simple remedies are a wonderful way to administer bitter-tasting medicinal herbs to reluctant children and adults alike. Sweet and delicious, syrups can be taken by the spoonful and make a lovely addition to teas, desserts, and bubbly beverages.

All syrups begin with a concentrated decoction, which is then cooked down and sweetened with either sugar or honey to help preserve the mix and add flavor. This process perfectly concentrates an herb's active constituents, making it great for treating upper respiratory infections.

Syrups prepared with honey are usually preferable to syrups prepared with sugar, as honey is naturally antibacterial and effective at soothing and coating sore throats. (Don't give honey to children younger than 2.)

If no preservatives are added to your syrup, it should last about two to three weeks. Add a few pinches of vitamin C powder to increase its refrigerated shelf life by one to two weeks.

Great For: Sore throats, upper respiratory infections, preventing and fighting colds and flu

Best Herbs for Syrups: Elderberry, echinacea, ginger, garlic, licorice, marshmallow root, peppermint, sage, thyme

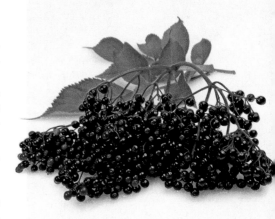

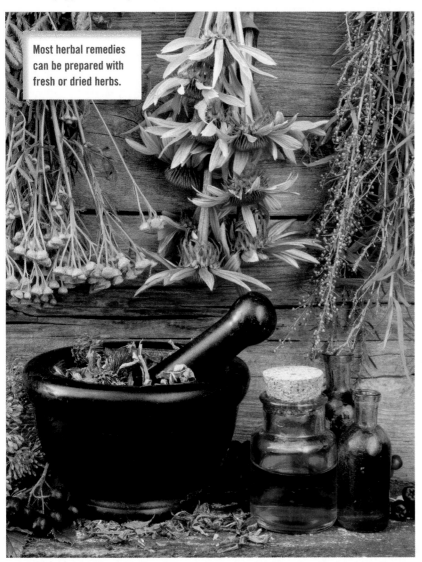

Most herbal remedies can be prepared with fresh or dried herbs.

Elderberry Syrup

This may be one of the better elderberry syrup recipes on the planet, according to herbalist Rosemary Gladstar. It's delicious enough to use for its flavor alone, but it's also helpful for warding off or speeding recovery from colds and flu, as elderberry has antiviral properties.

Be sure to cook elderberries thoroughly. Raw elderberry fruit, flowers, and leaves contain a chemical that produces cyanide, which can cause nausea and vomiting at high doses.

Ingredients
- 2 quarts fresh ripe elderberries
- ¼ cup warm water
- ¼ ounce freshly grated ginger root
- ½ teaspoon ground cloves
- Honey

Directions: Combine elderberries with water in a large soup pot and simmer until soft. Strain out pulp, reserving liquid. Discard solids and return liquid to pot.

Add ginger and cloves, and simmer uncovered until liquid reduces by about half. Pour juice into a measuring cup and note its volume, then return to pot. Add the same amount of honey as you have juice, and stir until thoroughly combined.

Let cool, then bottle. Store in the refrigerator and use within 12 weeks.

Take 1 to 2 tablespoons several times a day.

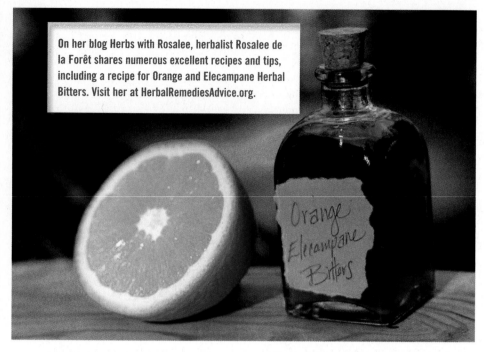

On her blog Herbs with Rosalee, herbalist Rosalee de la Forêt shares numerous excellent recipes and tips, including a recipe for Orange and Elecampane Herbal Bitters. Visit her at HerbalRemediesAdvice.org.

Bitters

Bitters have long been used to treat illness and flavor cocktails. Made of medicinal, bitter roots, barks, or leaves, bitters are primarily taken to enhance appetite and improve digestion. The theory is that the strong, acrid taste of bitters hitting the taste buds signals production of more saliva, acids, enzymes, hormones, bile, and so forth, in turn stimulating and improving the activity of the digestive organs as a whole. Bitters are also said to support liver function and boost metabolism.

To make this age-old remedy, tincture the fresh or dried digestive herbs of your choice with 100-proof vodka. Store the solution in a dark amber or cobalt bottle — use dropper bottles to make dosing easier. You can simply add drops directly to your tongue. Bitters can also be added to soda water or cocktails. To improve digestion, take about a teaspoon before or after dinner.

Great For: Stimulating digestion, increasing appetite, supporting metabolism and liver function

Best Herbs for Bitters: Angelica, bitter melon, chamomile, chicory, dandelion, gentian, ginger, orange peel

Dandy Tummy Bitters

This bitter-aromatic formula is perfect to have on hand during that next big feast. In addition to dandelion's bitterness, the aromatics from fennel, ginger, and orange help curb post-dessert bloat and can help relieve excess acid in the stomach, too.

Ingredients
- 2 parts dandelion root
- 1 part fennel seed
- ½ part ginger root
- ½ part orange peel
- 100-proof vodka

Directions: If tincturing fresh herbs, first clean them, then finely chop or grind them.

Fill ½ of a clean Mason jar with the mixture. If tincturing dried herbs, only fill ⅓ of the jar, as dried roots will expand.

Cover herbs with 100-proof vodka, filling to the top of the jar. Be sure your herb mixture is completely covered. Allow mixture to extract for 6 to 8 weeks, shaking often. Strain herbs with cheesecloth and squeeze any remaining liquid back into the extract.

Bottle liquid in amber dropper bottles and label with name, date, and parts used.

Recipe excerpted with permission from the Mountain Rose Blog (MountainRoseBlog.com) by Mountain Rose Herbs.

Elixirs

Elixirs are another tasty and traditional way to take your herbs. They are essentially sweetened tinctures that typically call on the healing powers of adaptogenic herbs. This useful group of herbs is well known for supporting the health of our adrenal systems, which manage our bodies' hormonal response to stress. These tonic herbs are useful for boosting energy, vitality, and possibly even longevity.

This sweet remedy is usually made with brandy, which is gentler on the stomach than other alcohols used for tincturing. It's also naturally warming, smooth, and tasty. Elixirs are typically made for sipping, as they are much more palatable than their tincture counterparts, and typically have a shelf life of about three years.

Great For: Enhancing energy and vitality, boosting immunity and overall wellness

Best Herbs for Elixirs: Astragalus, ashwagandha, damiana, fo-ti, ginger, ginseng, gotu kola, rhodiola, saw palmetto

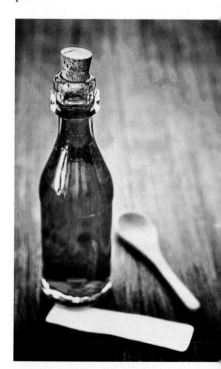

Being much more palatable than tinctures, elixirs are often made for sipping.

Long-Life Elixir

This herbal tonic builds strength and vitality. Although it can be used by both sexes, it was formulated specifically for men. You can use different herbs with other health benefits, different proportions, and even different flavoring agents—I've never followed the exact recipe twice myself. For each quart of tincture, use two good-sized, high-quality ginseng roots, or whatever you can afford. This strong herbal tonic will taste like a rich liqueur and is excellent for you. Serve it in a fine little goblet and sip it as an aperitif.

Damiana is not recommended for diabetics; pregnant or nursing women; or within two weeks of surgery. Fo-ti is not recommended for children; pregnant or nursing women; diabetics; those with liver disease; or within two weeks of surgery.

Ingredients

- 2 parts damiana leaf
- 2 parts fo-ti
- 2 parts ginger root
- 2 parts licorice
- 2 parts sassafras root bark
- 1 part astragalus
- 1 part Chinese star anise
- ¼ part saw palmetto berries
- Asian ginseng roots
  (2 per quart of elixir)
- Brandy
- Black cherry concentrate

Directions: Place herbs in a wide-mouth glass jar and cover with a good-quality brandy. Seal with a tight-fitting lid and let sit for 6 to 8 weeks—the longer the better.

Strain, discard herbs, and reserve liquid. To each cup of liquid, add ½ cup black cherry concentrate. Be sure this is fruit concentrate, not fruit juice, and do not add more than ½ cup per cup of tincture.

Shake well and rebottle.

I often put the whole ginseng roots back into the tincture, but they also can be sliced first.

A standard daily dose is about ⅛ cup.

Recipe adapted from Rosemary Gladstar's Herbal Recipes for Vibrant Health; used with permission of Storey Publishing. Available at MotherEarthNews.com/Store.

Vinegars

Although they are not as potent as alcohol-based tinctures, medicinal vinegars are an excellent choice for people with an intolerance to alcohol. Vinegars have been used for thousands of years to preserve foods, and, thanks to recent studies, we now know that vinegar offers a multitude of health benefits of its own. Apple cider vinegar, in particular, may be helpful in treating diabetes, high cholesterol, poor digestion, and minor skin ailments.

Extract nutritious herbs (fresh or dried) with this kitchen staple, and enjoy atop salads and veggies or drink diluted in tea or water. (Avoid direct contact with your teeth, as the acid content in vinegar could harm them.) Compared with alcohol-based tinctures, herbal vinegars have a shorter shelf life—about six months—and don't draw out as many beneficial components of a plant. However, vinegars excel at drawing out minerals and vitamins. As a general guide, take 1 tablespoon vinegar extract up to five times daily as needed.

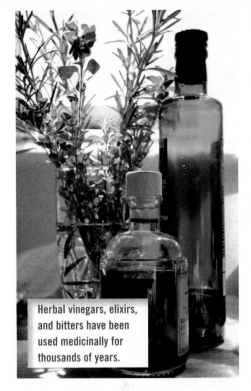

Herbal vinegars, elixirs, and bitters have been used medicinally for thousands of years.

Great For: Enhancing nutrition, fending off colds and flu, boosting immunity, lowering cholesterol, relieving arthritis, improving digestion

Best Herbs for Vinegars: Dandelion, elderberry, lavender, oregano, plantain, rosemary, sage, thyme, yellow dock 🌿

'Four Thieves' Healing Vinegar

According to French folklore, during the 17th century, this concoction of herbs and vinegar kept four thieves (grave robbers, actually) from contracting the dreaded black plague. It was said that by dousing face masks with this brew, the thieves were able to rob the graves and houses of the recently deceased without falling ill.

I believe it—these herbs are potent antivirals, anti-inflammatories, and immune-boosters. When you feel colds, flu, or (heaven forbid) the plague approaching, douse your salads and veggies in this (actually quite tasty) vinegar. You can also take it by the tablespoonful in warm water with a dash of honey and lemon.

Wormwood is not recommended for pregnant or nursing women, and could be problematic for those with a kidney disorder, a seizure disorder, porphyria, or a ragweed allergy.

Ingredients

- 2 tablespoons dried rosemary
- 2 tablespoons dried sage
- 2 tablespoons dried lavender
- 2 tablespoons dried wormwood
- 2 tablespoons dried peppermint
- 1 quart raw, organic apple cider vinegar
- 2 tablespoons fresh garlic, chopped

Directions: In a clean, quart-size glass jar, combine the first 6 ingredients. Cover and steep in a cool dark place for about 2 weeks, shaking daily.

Strain out herbs and return vinegar to jar. Add garlic and cover. Let steep for a few days more and strain again.

Store in the fridge for up to 6 months.

Recipe excerpted from Herbal Goddess by Amy Jirsa; used with permission of Storey Publishing. Available at MotherEarthNews.com/Store.

Tea Time

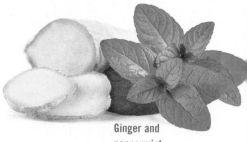

Ginger and peppermint

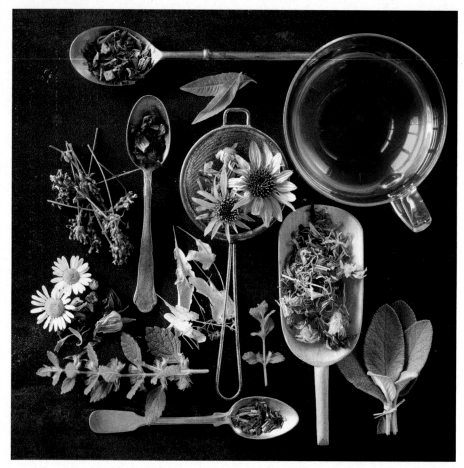

Try these easy herbal teas for 10 common health problems.

By *Mother Earth News* editors

Steaming, delicious herbal tea can do more for us than act as an afternoon pick-me-up. A wide variety of herbs have healing applications, and they can be administered as a lovely cup of tea. From classic calming herbs such as lavender and chamomile to garden standbys such as rosehips and sage—and even plants known as weeds such as dandelion—many herbs can help us feel better on a regular basis.

1. Chamomile for Anxiety

Although chamomile is a gentle healer, it's still highly effective. This yellow daisylike flower is a popular medicine among herbalists, as it's known to treat a variety of ailments. The flowers contain high amounts of the volatile oil azulene, which has anti-inflammatory properties. Chamomile is also a popular remedy to reduce anxiety and quiet the mind for sleep.

To Make Tea: Gather 1 teaspoon dried or 2 teaspoons fresh chamomile flowers and steep in 1 cup boiling water for 15 to 20 minutes. The longer it steeps, the more bitter it will taste.

2. Lavender for Sleep Problems

A beautiful and fragrant addition to any garden, lavender has profound relaxing, calming, and uplifting effects. A number of studies have shown this violet beauty to help slow the activity of the nervous system, improve sleep quality, promote relaxation, and lift mood. It's most popular as an aromatherapy aid, where it's used in inhalation therapy to treat headaches and reduce stress, as well as a topical aid where its antifungal actions come in handy. But it also makes a wonderful healing tea.

To Make Tea: Harvest lavender flowers when the buds are just starting to open for the highest quality, according to *Rosemary Gladstar's Medicinal Herbs*. Steep 4 teaspoons fresh lavender buds in 1 cup boiling water for 10 minutes, then enjoy.

3. Peppermint for Indigestion

Renewing, refreshing, and energizing peppermint is the perfect herbal pick-me-up. It's renowned as a digestive aid—use this aromatic herb to relieve nausea and gas. Several studies have shown it to be effective at treating symptoms of indigestion and irritable bowel syndrome. Its main active agent, menthol, also works as a decongestant and may help loosen phlegm and break up coughs during cold and flu season.

To Make Tea: Steep 1 teaspoon dried peppermint leaves in 1 cup boiling water for 10 minutes. Drink four to five times per day between meals.

4. Ginger for Nausea

We naturally associate this pungent herb with winter, thanks to its warming properties. In addition to helping boost circulation during cold weather, the fragrant root is also known to soothe upset stomachs and help ease nausea in general, especially from motion sickness. It is also known to help with the nausea pregnant women can experience.

To Make Tea: Steep three to five thin slices of ginger root in boiling water for three minutes; strain. You can also grate the ginger root into a tea ball; steep for three minutes.

5. Raspberry for Menstrual Cramps

Raspberry leaf is naturally rich in nutrients, including magnesium, potassium, iron, and B vitamins. Thanks to its unique components, it's perfect for the female reproductive system. Use it to soothe menstrual cramps, as it can strengthen the uterus and pelvic muscles. Its astringent properties also make it wonderful for alleviating motion sickness and dispelling diarrhea. It helps "dry up" the mucous membrane of the intestine. **Note:** Raspberry leaf should not be taken during pregnancy.

To Make Tea: Steep 1 tablespoon dried raspberry leaf in 8 ounces boiling water for at least five minutes. If using fresh leaves, Dr. Andrew Weil suggested first picking leaves off their brambles, hanging them to dry, then steeping them in boiling water. Drink up to 6 cups a day for acute problems as needed.

6. Lemon Balm for Anxiety

Lemon balm is renowned for its treatment of anxiety. It's also known as a natural relaxation aid. Researchers reported finding that lemon balm helped nix anxiety in the journal *Phytotherapy Research*. The herb has also been shown to inhibit viruses, such as the herpes virus that causes cold sores and even HIV. It also can help fight headaches and reduce insomnia.

To Make Tea: Steep 1 to 2 teaspoons of dried lemon balm per cup of boiled water. Let steep until it's cool enough to drink.

7. Basil for Bad Breath

Basil is an excellent source of vitamins A and K, plus a good source of vitamin C and manganese. It is also rich in antioxidants and has antibacterial properties. Research showed the natural volatile oils in basil inhibited multiple drug-resistant strains of *E. coli* bacteria. Basil also makes an absolutely delightful breath refresher.

To Make Tea: Steep 2 teaspoons dried basil leaves in 1 cup boiling water for 20 minutes. Strain and sweeten, if desired.

8. Sage for Sore Throats

This garden staple is easy to grow, beautiful in the garden and has the benefit of making a throat-soothing tea. Its antimicrobial properties help you fight off colds, as well as treat the accompanying symptoms such as a sore throat. **Note:** Avoid using sage if you have epilepsy.

To Make Tea: Combine 3 teaspoons dried sage leaves or 10 fresh sage leaves and 1 cup boiling water. Let steep five minutes. Then strain and enjoy.

9. Rosehips to Boost Immunity

Rose bushes that are not deadheaded (removing dead flower heads to encourage more blooming) by a gardener develop rosehips, which are full of seeds and sometimes pulp. They make a wonderful source of immune-boosting vitamin C and have even been used in the past to treat scurvy. In fact, by volume, rosehips contain about 20 times the vitamin C as oranges.

To Make Tea: Combine 4 tablespoons whole dried rosehips with 4 cups water in a saucepan. Cover, bring to a boil, then simmer for five minutes. Strain into a teapot, and drink when sufficiently cool.

10. Dandelion for Bone Health

Although it's generally regarded as a weed, this plant is packed with essential minerals such as iron, potassium, and beta-carotene, plus vitamins A, C, and D.

Combined with a physically active lifestyle, the powerful punch of vitamin D in dandelion tea can help build strong bones and ward off osteoporosis. (To read more about this, visit MotherEarth News.com/Build-Strong-Bones.) The young, delicate leaves are also delicious in a salad or steamed with garlic and chili pepper flakes.

To Make Tea: Boil 1 quart water. Turn off heat and add 4 tablespoons dandelion leaf. Cover and steep 30 to 60 minutes, then strain. 🌿

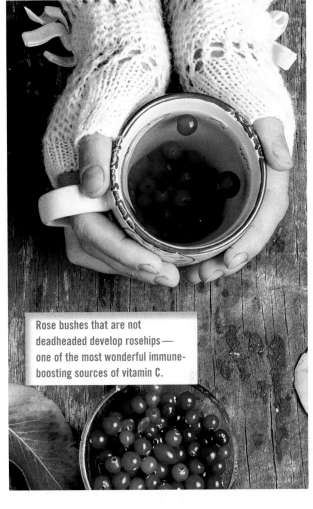

Rose bushes that are not deadheaded develop rosehips — one of the most wonderful immune-boosting sources of vitamin C.

Heal Like an
EGYPTIAN

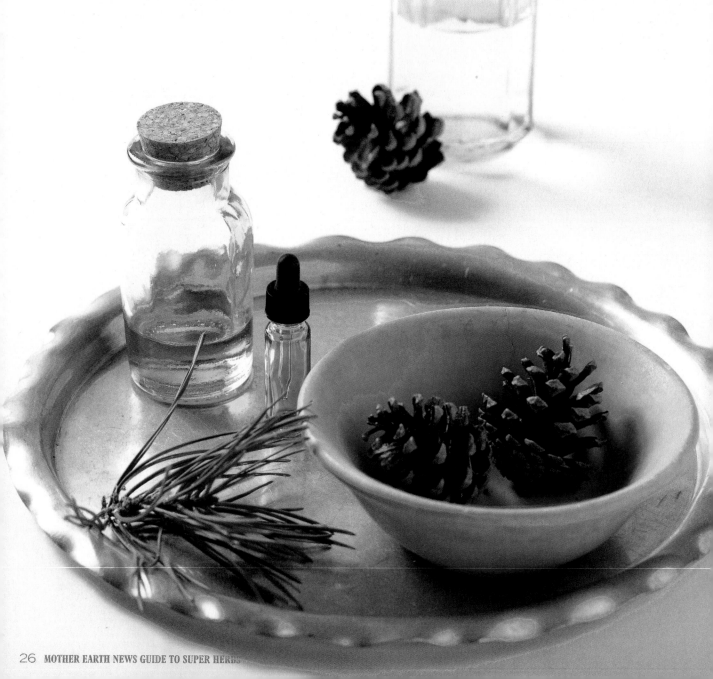

Free yourself from pain, fatigue, and more with the ancient herbal art of aromatherapy.

By Laurel Vukovic

Essential oils have been a precious commodity throughout history, and have been used extensively in India, China, the Middle East, and Europe. The Egyptians were skilled in using essential oils and employed fragrances such as cedarwood, frankincense, myrrh, and juniper in cosmetics, as well as using them for healing and embalming.

The Greeks enthusiastically adopted the use of essential oils from the Egyptians, perfuming their food and drink in addition to their bodies and clothing. The famed Greek physician Hippocrates had a delightful prescription for longevity: a daily soak in a scented bath, followed by an aromatherapy massage. He might have been onto something. Researchers today are finding essential oils to have measurable effects on the body and emotions.

What are Essential Oils?

Essential oils give many flowers, herbs, spices, and fruits their characteristic scents. The pungent scent of peppermint, the spicy aroma of cloves, and the sweet fragrance of jasmine are all the result of the plants' essential oils. Plants produce these fragrant oils to stimulate growth and reproduction, to attract beneficial insects and discourage harmful ones, and to protect the plant from diseases. Some of these properties are useful for us, too. For example, citronella, cedarwood, and lemongrass are essential components of natural insect repellents, and eucalyptus and thyme are added to common household products such as disinfectants and mouthwashes.

Aromatic oils are found in all parts of plants. Peel an orange and you've released the abundant essential oils found in its skin. But not all essential oils are so easily obtained. Most require distillation, a process of heating the plant in water, capturing the steam, and separating the droplets of essential oil from the steam as it condenses. The result is a highly concentrated oil that captures the fragrance of the plant. It takes about 1 ton of rose petals (close to 60,000 roses) to produce just 1 ounce of rose oil.

The Healing Properties of Essential Oils

As ancient people knew, the benefits of essential oils go far beyond their pleasing aromas. These concentrated plant essences retain the healing properties of the herbs and flowers from which they are distilled, and can be used for treating both physical and psychological disorders.

When essential oils are inhaled or applied to the skin, the aromatic molecules enter the bloodstream and are circulated throughout the body. For this reason they can be used for a variety of physical conditions, from fighting respiratory infections to relieving digestive upsets, headaches, and PMS.

The effects of essential oils on the emotions are the result of a different physiological pathway. Chemicals in the air stimulate olfactory cells in the nose, which relay the information to the brain, where smell is perceived. The olfactory nerve pathways are tied in with the brain's limbic area, the seat of our emotions, memories, intuition and sexual response. That's why the sense of smell is the most influential trigger of memories and emotions.

It is important to choose fragrances that appeal to you because scents evoke vivid memories and emotions. For example, although lavender is regarded as an excellent scent for easing tension, if you associate it with your punitive second-grade teacher who used lavender soap, then it's not likely to make you feel relaxed.

Scientific Support for Aromatherapy

Researchers throughout the world are proving what the ancients knew: Essential oils have powerful effects on the mind and body. John Steele, an aromatic consultant in California, and Robert

Energizing Essential Oils

- Basil (*Ocimum basilicum*)
- Bergamot (*Citrus ×aurantium*)
- Eucalyptus (*Eucalyptus globulus*)
- Grapefruit (*Citrus ×paradisi*)
- Lemon (*Citrus ×limon*)
- Lime (*Citrus ×aurantiifolia*)
- Peppermint (*Mentha ×piperita*)
- Rosemary (*Rosmarinus officinalis*)
- Sweet orange (*Citrus ×sinensis*)

Relaxing Essential Oils

- German chamomile (*Matricaria chamomilla*)
- Clary sage (*Salvia sclarea*)
- Frankincense (*Boswellia sacra*)
- Geranium (*Pelargonium graveolens*)
- Jasmine (*Jasminum officinale*)
- Lavender (*Lavandula angustifolia*)
- Marjoram (*Origanum majorana*)
- Neroli (*Citrus ×aurantium*)
- Patchouli (*Pogostemon cablin*)
- Rose (*Rosa* spp.)
- Sandalwood (*Santalum album*)
- Ylang ylang (*Cananga odorata*)

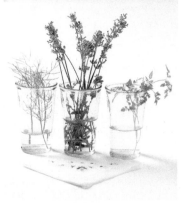

Tisserand, a leading British aromatherapist, have studied the effects of essential oils on brain wave patterns. They've shown that beta brain waves, which indicate a state of heightened awareness, are increased when stimulating oils such as black pepper, rosemary, or basil are inhaled. Calming oils such as neroli, jasmine, lavender, and rose produce more alpha and theta brain waves, indicating relaxation and well-being.

In other studies, researchers at Memorial Sloan-Kettering Cancer Center in New York found that patients who were exposed to the scent of heliotrope (a vanilla-like fragrance) while undergoing diagnostic medical tests were significantly less anxious. A Duke University Hospital study found that the daily use of fragrance dramatically improved the mood of women at midlife. And in a study reported in the British medical journal *Lancet*, elderly patients suffering from insomnia found that the aroma of lavender helped them fall asleep quicker and sleep longer than did prescription sedatives.

How to Use Essential Oils

Baths: Add 3 to 10 drops of essential oil (or of a combination of essential oils) to a bathtub of warm water. To prevent possible skin irritation, first dilute the essential oil in 1 teaspoon of vegetable oil or liquid soap. You can also mix 10 drops of essential oil with 1 cup of baking soda in a plastic container, shake well, then add to the bathtub. Stir the water with your hand to dissolve the mixture. Soak for 10 to 20 minutes.

Simple inhalation: Place 1 drop of essential oil onto a handkerchief or tissue; inhale as desired. Depending on the oil used, this can allay stress, improve concentration, or clear the sinuses.

Steam inhalation: Pour 2 quarts of boiling water into a heatproof bowl. Add 3 drops of essential oil. Make a tent over your head and the bowl with a large bath towel. Inhale the fragrant steam for 10 minutes, taking care to not burn yourself with the steam. This is excellent for relieving sinus congestion, colds, and sore throat, and for deep-cleansing the skin.

Air freshener: Add 6 drops of essential oil to 1 cup of water in a clean spray bottle. Shake well and use as you would any air freshener. To prevent staining, avoid spraying onto wood surfaces or upholstered furniture. This neutralizes odors and provides a calming or energizing influence, depending on the oils used.

Use Essential Oils Safely

- In general, don't use essential oils undiluted on your skin. However, unless your skin is especially sensitive, you may discover that some essential oils are safe to apply directly. For example, lavender can be used for insect bites or burns; tea tree oil can be dabbed on pimples; and sandalwood, rose, or ylang ylang can be applied as perfume oils.
- Do not take essential oils internally without the guidance of a qualified aromatherapy practitioner.
- Keep essential oils away from your eyes.
- Avoid oils that can cause photosensitivity: Bergamot (unless it is labeled as bergapten-free), lemon, lime, and orange essential oils can all cause uneven skin pigmentation if used within four hours of exposure to sunlight.
- Keep essential oils out of the reach of children. When using essential oils for children, use only nontoxic and nonirritating oils such as lavender and chamomile. Use 1 drop of essential oil in a bath or in 1 teaspoon of massage oil for babies up to 12 months; one-third of the adult dosage for children 1 to 5 years old; and one-half of the adult dosage for children up to the age of 12.
- Use essential oils with caution during pregnancy. In general, use half of the usual adult dosage while pregnant and stick with nonstimulating oils such as chamomile, frankincense, lavender, geranium, grapefruit, neroli, rose, and sandalwood. 🌿

Laurel Vukovic writes about herbs and natural healing from her home in southern Oregon. She is the author of *Herbal Healing Secrets for Women* (Prentice Hall, 2000).

Essential Oil Primer

Lift your spirits with the enticing aromas of essential oils.

Herb	Latin name	Uses
Basil	(*Ocimum basilicum*)	Basil calms nerves, improves mood, and sharpens senses.
Bergamot	(*Citrus xaurantium*)	Bergamot relieves anxiety and depression. It has calming and uplifting qualities.
Chamomile, Roman	(*Chamaemelum nobile*)	Chamomile is excellent for calming the nerves and relaxing stress, but is an expensive essential oil.
Clary sage	(*Salvia sclarea*)	Clary sage gives a sense of well-being and optimism.
Eucalyptus	(*Eucalyptus globulus*)	Eucalyptus dispels mental exhaustion and stimulates concentration.
Geranium	(*Pelargonium graveolens*)	Geranium eases nervous tension and enhances feelings of love and romance.
Ginger	(*Zingiber officinale*)	Ginger warms the emotions, uplifts the spirit, and helps aid concentration and memory retention.
Grapefruit	(*Citrus xparadisi*)	Grapefruit is excellent for lifting depression and giving a sense of well-being.
Lavender	(*Lavandula angustifolia*)	Lavender is widely known for stress relief and its wonderful calming effect. It aids in sleep for young and old alike.
Lemon	(*Citrus xlimon*)	Lemon rejuvenates the tired mind and spirit. It aids in concentration and promotes clear thinking.
Marjoram	(*Origanum majorana*)	Sweet marjoram has calming qualities and helps relieve stress, headaches, and irritability. Its soothing fragrance aids in sleep.
Patchouli	(*Pogostemon cablin*)	Patchouli gives a sense of peace, calm, love, and well-being.
Peppermint	(*Mentha xpiperita*)	Peppermint is well-known for its stimulating and fatigue-relieving properties. It perks up the brain and helps in concentration.
Rosemary	(*Rosmarinus officinalis*)	Rosemary clears and energizes the senses, and is a great pick-me-up after a tiring day. It aids in concentration and memory.
Sandalwood	(*Santalum album*)	Sandalwood relieves stress and tension, and helps in meditation. For centuries it has been used as an aphrodisiac.
Thyme	(*Thymus vulgaris*)	Thyme revives and stimulates the senses. It helps improve memory and concentration.
Ylang ylang	(*Cananga odorata*)	Ylang ylang is used to lower high blood pressure and dispel depression. It creates a sense of euphoria, and its sweet fragrance promotes romance.

Body-Care Basics

Avoid toxic chemicals and ramp up your self-reliance by trying these simple recipes for basic body-care products.

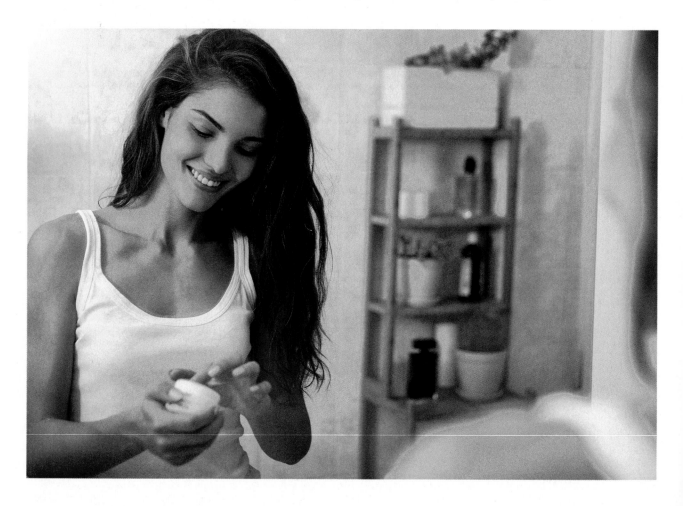

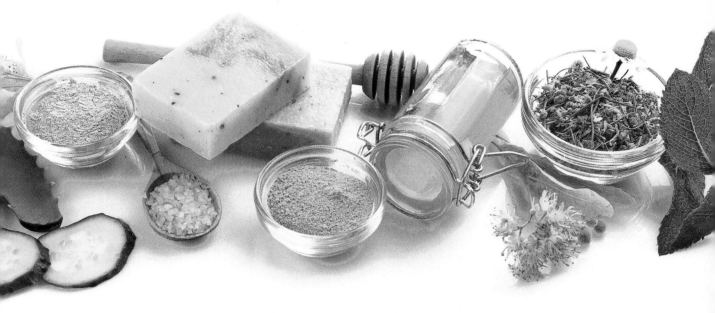

By Michelle Schoffro Cook

The huge array of everyday body-care products found on pharmacy and grocery store shelves contains thousands of chemicals—some of them known carcinogens, others potent endocrine disruptors, and most entirely untested. Many of these chemicals can be absorbed into our bodies through our skin and mouth. The good news is that these potentially harmful chemicals leave our bodies quickly. In one recent study by California researchers, girls between ages 14 and 18 had lower urinary concentrations of some chemicals (including triclosan, some types of parabens, and phthalates) after just three days without using cosmetics containing these substances.

Although many safer options exist (to find them, consult the Environmental Working Group's Skin Deep Database), making our own body-care products is a surefire way to eliminate these sources of unwanted toxins. And making our own cosmetics offers an added bonus: It's a great way to add more healing herbs into our lives.

Fortunately making our own products with natural ingredients is much easier than you might think. Although most commercial body-care products contain a slew of ingredients, homemade versions can often be made with just a handful of natural items. In this article, I've highlighted some of the worst chemicals to avoid, and the simple ways to make your own luxurious, pleasurable replacements.

Creams & Lotions

Commercial Culprits: BHA and BHT

The full names of these chemicals are butylated hydroxyanisole and butylated hydroxytoluene. The first is a suspected endocrine disruptor and carcinogen. The second is a suspected carcinogen that may also be linked with developmental problems.

Superior Herbal Ingredients: Horsetail and Yarrow

Horsetail and yarrow both support healthy skin and help to heal damaged skin and wounds. Yarrow helps with healing wounds and blemishes, and it's been shown to significantly reduce the visibility of wrinkles and pores.

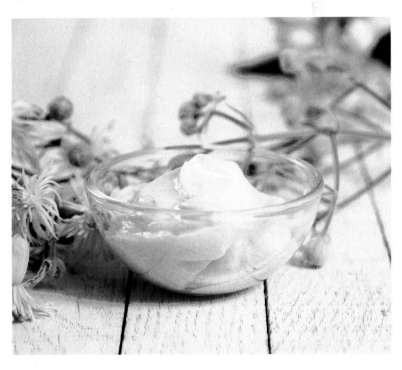

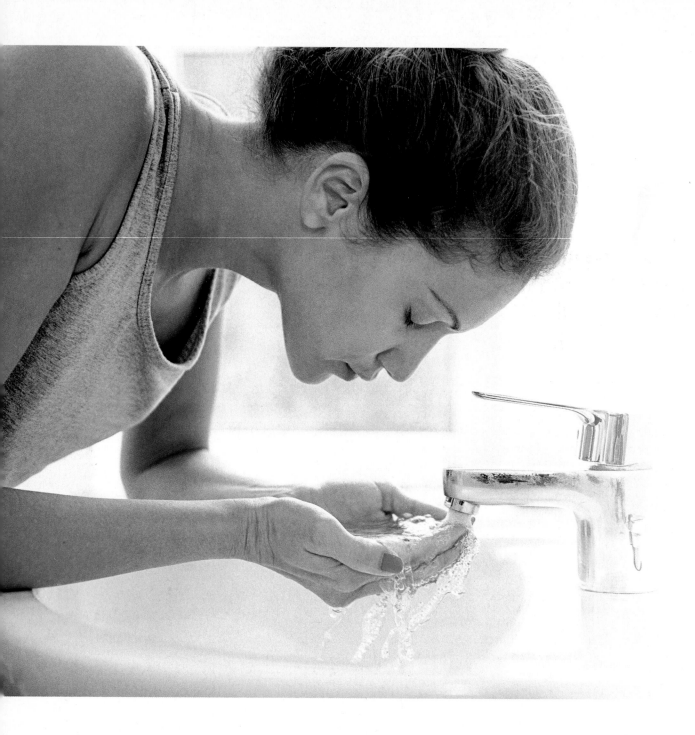

Facial Toners

Commercial Culprit: Acetone

This harsh ingredient is commonly found in facial toners, even though it can irritate the skin and may be linked with neurotoxicity.

Superior Herbal Ingredient: Yarrow

According to the *International Journal of Cosmetic Science*, an extract of yarrow applied to the skin significantly reduced the visibility of wrinkles and pores, compared with a placebo and glycolic acid products. Glycolic acid is a substance frequently added to antiwrinkle creams to help remove dead skin cells and give skin a fresher look. Don't be surprised if you start seeing yarrow extracts used in the cosmetics industry in the future.

Recipes

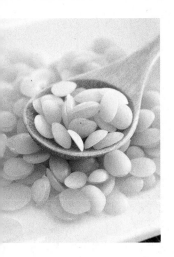

Horsetail Skin-Healing Lotion

This soothing, all-purpose lotion can be used daily for a wide variety of skin conditions. **Makes about 2 cups.**

Ingredients
- 1 cup purified water
- 2 teaspoons dried horsetail, or 4 teaspoons fresh
- ¾ cup sweet almond or apricot kernel oil
- 2 tablespoons shaved beeswax

Directions: Boil water and pour over herb. Cover and let mixture brew for 10 to 20 minutes. Strain out herb, reserving herbal infusion.

Pour oil into a glass measuring cup and add beeswax. Set it in a saucepan of water that reaches about halfway up the side of the glass container. Heat mixture on stove over low heat until beeswax dissolves, then immediately remove pan from heat. Allow it to cool for a minute or two, but not longer, as beeswax will begin to harden.

Pour herbal infusion into blender and begin blending on high speed with lid on (with a hole left in the lid for pouring the beeswax-oil mixture). Slowly pour oil-beeswax mixture into the water. It will begin to thicken after about ¾ of the oil has been incorporated. Continue adding oil until you've incorporated all of it.

Immediately pour lotion into jars. Use a spatula to remove any remaining lotion from the blender. Because it's free of preservatives, it's best to store this lotion in the fridge, where it will last about 3 months.

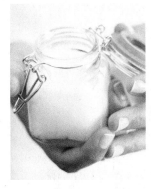

Yarrow Antiwrinkle Skin Refresher Cream

Why use wrinkle creams that are full of toxic chemicals and cost a fortune, when you can make your own that are much better for your skin and overall health? Some people experience skin irritation from yarrow, so it's a good idea to test this cream on an inconspicuous area such as the inside of your wrist, and wait at least 48 hours before using on your face. **Makes about 1¾ cups.**

Ingredients
- 2 teaspoons dried yarrow flowers and leaves, or 4 teaspoons fresh

- 1 cup water
- ¾ cup sweet almond oil or apricot kernel oil
- 2 tablespoons shaved beeswax

Directions: Boil water and pour it over yarrow. Cover mixture and let brew for 10 to 20 minutes. Strain out yarrow, reserving yarrow-infused water. Set aside.

Pour oil into a glass measuring cup and add beeswax. Set measuring cup in a saucepan of water that reaches about halfway up the side of the measuring cup. Heat mixture until beeswax melts, then immediately remove measuring cup from heat. Allow to cool for a minute or two, but not longer, as the beeswax will begin to harden.

Pour yarrow-infused water into a blender, cover, and begin blending on high speed. With blender running, slowly pour beeswax mixture through the hole in the blender lid. The mixture will begin to thicken after about ¾ of the beeswax has been incorporated.

Once beeswax is fully blended, immediately pour lotion into a 16-ounce glass jar or two 8-ounce glass jars. Use a spatula to remove any remaining cream from the blender. The cream lasts about 3 months and is best kept in the refrigerator.

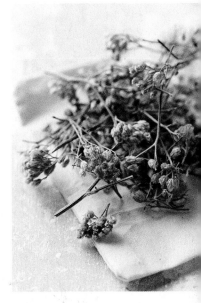

Yarrow Facial Toner

It's easy to make a facial toner with yarrow that cleanses the skin, tightens the pores, and alleviates oily patches, while also helping minimize the appearance of wrinkles.

Ingredients
- 1 cup water, boiled
- 2 teaspoons dried yarrow
- 1 tablespoon witch hazel

Directions: Pour boiled water over yarrow and let steep for at least 15 minutes. Let cool.

Add witch hazel and pour mixture into a spray bottle. Spritz toner on skin or pour a small amount onto a cotton ball and apply to skin. The toner will last for up to 1 month in the refrigerator.

Hair Conditioner

Commercial Culprits: Parabens

Parabens are xenoestrogens (chemicals that mimic estrogen in the body) that may be linked with breast cancer.

Superior Herbal Ingredient: Rosemary

Not only does rosemary smell great, but it may help reduce testosterone levels below the skin. Excessive testosterone can cause hair thinning in men and women. In an article published in the journal *Phytotherapy Research*, scientists found that applying an extract made of rosemary improved hair regrowth in animals affected by excess testosterone. Scientists found that the rosemary extract appears to block dihydrotestosterone, a more potent form of testosterone, from binding to receptor sites.

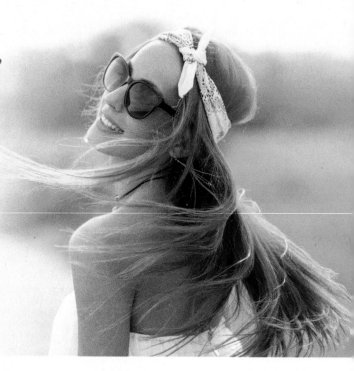

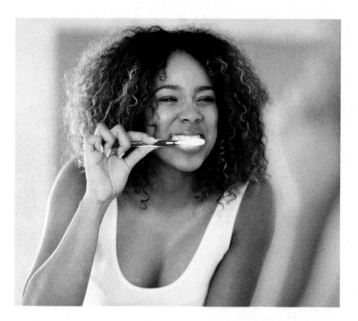

Toothpaste

Commercial Culprit: Triclosan

Triclosan is a suspected endocrine disruptor and a well-known antibiotic known to contribute to the rise of antibiotic-resistant pathogens. The best-selling brand Colgate Total is among the only commercial toothpastes to contain triclosan.

Superior Herbal Ingredients: Peppermint and Myrrh Essential Oils

These oils offer natural antibacterial properties. Peppermint essential oil helps freshen breath, kill bacteria, and clear sinuses. Myrrh oil is antibacterial and antifungal.

Deodorant

Commercial Culprits: Triclosan and "Fragrance"

As previously mentioned, triclosan is an endocrine disruptor and contributor to antibiotic resistance. Fragrance, also listed as "parfum" on labels, can contain a mix of many ingredients that may have associated health concerns, none of which must be labeled because they are considered proprietary.

Superior Herbal Ingredient: Tea Tree Essential Oil

Tea tree is known for cleansing the skin, for boosting immune function, and for its antibacterial properties, when applied topically. That makes it the perfect natural ingredient for making deodorant or other skin-care products. The Australian aboriginal people have used this herb for centuries.

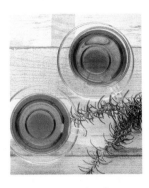

Rosemary Hair Rinse

This is a great natural hair rinse and leave-in conditioner for all hair types. If you're interested in promoting hair growth, apply the tonic to the scalp daily for at least a couple of months. Simply pour over your scalp and leave it in your hair as it dries, or spritz clean, towel-dried hair daily, ensuring that you spritz the scalp.

Ingredients
- 1 quart water
- 2 to 3 (6-inch) sprigs fresh rosemary

Directions: In a pot, bring water to a boil. Turn off heat, add rosemary. Cover with a lid. Allow to sit for 20 minutes.

Allow liquid to cool, then remove rosemary and pour into a bottle. Store hair tonic in the fridge for up to a week.

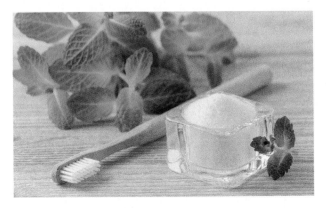

Natural Tooth Powder

This powder combines the power of two essential oils with the cleaning power of baking soda. **Makes ½ cup.**

Ingredients
- ½ cup baking soda
- 10 drops peppermint essential oil
- 5 drops myrrh essential oil (optional)

Directions: Mix ingredients in a jar with a lid, cover, and shake vigorously.

Use a small amount on a damp toothbrush, as you use toothpaste.

All-Natural Deodorant

My friend Kim, creator of natural wellness products, shared this recipe for her favorite natural deodorant.

Ingredients
- 6 tablespoons coconut oil
- 4 tablespoons shea butter
- 2 tablespoons beeswax
- 2 tablespoons almond oil
- 3 tablespoons arrowroot powder
- 3 tablespoons diatomaceous earth (optional)

100% of 20 teens in an Environmental Working Group study had methylparaben & propylparaben in their urine.

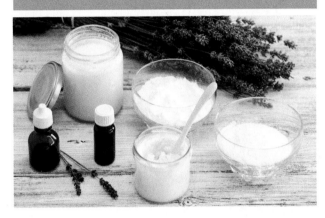

- 5 drops vitamin E oil
- 50 drops essential oils such as tea tree, thyme, lavender, or rosemary

Directions: Melt coconut oil, shea butter, and beeswax in a small pot over low heat until just melted, stirring constantly.

Add almond oil and stir to combine. Remove from heat and add arrowroot and diatomaceous earth, if using. Mix well. Add vitamin E oil and essential oils, and stir to combine.

Immediately pour into a glass jar or a deodorant tube (found in many health-food and craft stores) and let sit

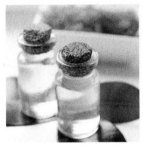

undisturbed until it hardens, about 4 hours. This deodorant does not need refrigeration. If using a glass jar, you can line it with cheesecloth so it will be easier to remove after it sets.

Recipes adapted with permission from Be Your Own Herbalist *by Michelle Schoffro Cook, PhD, DNM.*

Michelle Schoffro Cook is the international best-selling author of *Be Your Own Herbalist* (New World Library), *60 Seconds to Slim* (Rodale), and *The Probiotic Promise* (DaCapo). All are available at MotherEarthNews.com/Store. Visit DrMichelleCook.com and WorldsHealthiestDiet.com to learn more about her work.

Medicines
in Your Spice Rack

Get back to basics with proven home remedies available in your kitchen cupboard.

By Amy Mayfield

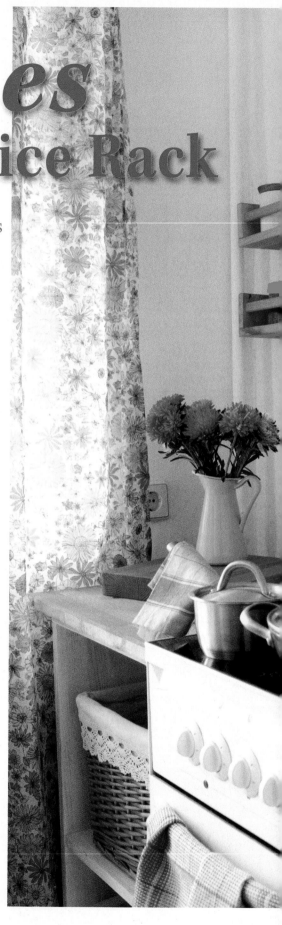

In this age of conflicting research, fancy (and expensive) supplements, and endless dialog about what we should do for our health, returning to the basics can be quite refreshing. After all, you can find some of the most effective herbal medicines right in your kitchen.

Culinary herbs such as basil, dill, and oregano all are great for your health — they're high in antioxidants and have carminative properties, meaning they enhance digestion and help relieve gas and bloating. But other herbs have been shown to have powerful health benefits, too, ranging from lowering cholesterol to smoothing out blood sugar levels. Here's a guide to several of the herbal superstars you likely have sitting in your spice rack, ready to boost the flavor and health factor of your meals.

Garlic: Curb Cholesterol, Prevent Cancer

One of the most revered medicines in history, garlic is a powerful healer with antiviral and antibacterial properties. It was a favorite of the ancient Egyptians who used the herb to prevent illness and even increase strength and endurance.

Modern research shows garlic can help lower cholesterol. In a study conducted at Penn State University and published in 2000, researchers gave either garlic or a placebo to men with high cholesterol. At the end of the study, the garlic group averaged a 7 percent drop in total cholesterol levels. Although some studies (widely reported in the mainstream media) have shown garlic to be ineffective against high cholesterol and heart disease, most studies do show a positive effect. That being said, garlic is not as powerful as statin drugs. If your cholesterol is high and unresponsive to healthy lifestyle changes, seek the advice of a medical professional.

In studies, garlic also has been shown to improve ulcers; lower the risk of heart attack and stroke; prevent cancer; reduce blood sugar levels; and more.

Taking garlic: Most herbalists recommend taking the equivalent of about one clove of raw or lightly cooked garlic a day. Garlic supplements (brands like Kyolic and Kwai) also are effective; follow manufacturers' dosage suggestions.

Safety concerns: Garlic (especially raw) can irritate the stomach. It also can impair blood clotting. Do not take it in large amounts if you

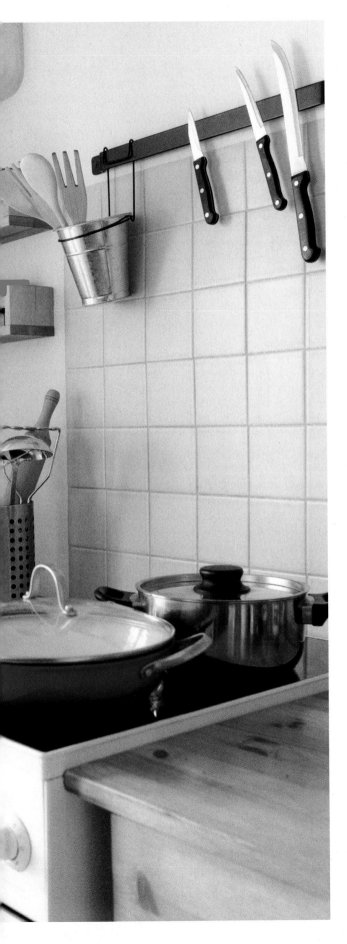

have a clotting disorder, and discontinue use two weeks before any scheduled surgery.

Turmeric: A Multitude of Uses

A standout in traditional Indian medicine (Ayurveda), turmeric is a brightly colored herb with a multitude of uses. In the U.S., it's best known as the source for mustard's bright-yellow color and as a key ingredient in curry powder. But turmeric's active constituent, curcumin, is a powerful healer. Herbalists recommend the herb for its potent anti-oxidant properties; for its liver-protective and detoxifying effects; to ease the pain of inflammatory joint conditions; and for its promising anti-cancer potential.

Taking turmeric: Use turmeric liberally in cooking: add it to soups, sauces, and vegetables such as green beans. When taking supplements, follow label directions. Generally, herbalists recommend about 1 gram of turmeric daily for maintenance and up to 30 grams for acute conditions.

Safety concerns: When taken in medicinal doses, turmeric can increase the blood-thinning effects of drugs such as aspirin and warfarin. Consult your physician if you take blood thinners and want to use turmeric. (There's no cause for alarm when enjoying turmeric for culinary uses.)

Settle Your Stomach with Tasty Ginger

Ginger is just about the most effective remedy around for settling a nauseous stomach, and research backs its effectiveness for relieving motion sickness and morning sickness. When Australian researchers gave 120 pregnant women either a placebo or a capsule with 1.5 grams of ginger powder, the ginger group experienced significantly less nausea, and the results were almost immediate. Ginger also is a warming herb that stimulates blood flow, which is beneficial for those with poor circulation. It can also shorten the duration of a cold or flu.

Taking ginger: Ginger generally is safe to take in fairly large amounts. Try a tea made with 2 teaspoons of fresh grated or chopped ginger root per cup of boiling water; a capsule with 1,000 to 1,500 mg of powdered ginger; or ginger ale that contains real ginger such as Reed's.

Safety concerns: Some people experience heartburn when using ginger, but overall it is a very safe herb. Pregnant women should avoid drinking more than three cups of ginger tea daily.

Web Extras

Discover the everyday healing power of flavorful culinary herbs. Visit MotherEarthNews.com/Healing-Power-Of-Culinary-Herbs for even more flavorful recipes made with delicious, medicinal herbs, including a Carrot and Ginger Energizer Smoothie, Salsa Verde, and Turmeric Yogurt Soup.

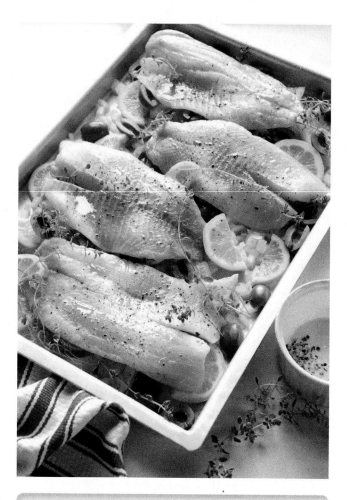

Potent Peppermint

A great-smelling herb with a long history of use as a stomach soother, peppermint is a good choice if you suffer from indigestion. In particular, it relaxes the intestinal tract and relieves painful gas. It also is helpful for easing nausea, heartburn, headaches, morning sickness, and even irritable bowel syndrome. (For IBS, it's most often taken in enteric-coated capsules.)

Taking peppermint: Try a cup of peppermint tea made with 1 teaspoon dried leaves or 1 tablespoon fresh leaves per cup of boiling water; steep 10 minutes, then strain and drink. Sweeten with honey, if desired. For enteric-coated capsules, follow label directions.

Safety concerns: Although there are many ways to use peppermint essential oil, never take it internally.

The Cozy Spice That's Great for Diabetics

The aroma of cinnamon conjures up cozy memories of warm fires and fresh-baked cookies—it's a favorite for many of us. A 2005 study published in the journal *Phytotherapy Research* revealed that cinnamon might be an effective treatment for diabetes. In the study, researchers gave 60 type 2 diabetics a placebo or cinnamon capsules (in dosages of 1, 3, or 6 grams daily). Six weeks later, diabetics taking all three cinnamon doses experienced reduced blood sugar (by 18 to 29 percent).

Cinnamon also has a long history of use as a stomach soother and digestive aid. The spice enhances the activity of trypsin, an enzyme that breaks down proteins in the small intestine; cinnamon also accelerates the breakdown of fats.

Taking cinnamon: To make cinnamon tea, pour 1 cup boiling water over ½ teaspoon ground cinnamon in a muslin bag. Steep, covered, for 10 minutes. Drink up to three cups daily.

Safety concerns: Cinnamon can cause rashes in sensitive individuals. Do not give cinnamon tea to children younger than 2.

Thyme: Terrific for Taming Coughs

Delicious thyme, a mint family member well-known in French cuisine, is a great choice if you're suffering from a cough, mucus congestion, sore throat, or bronchitis. Research has shown that the herb's expectorant (phlegm-loosening) properties can be attributed to two constituents: thymol and carvacrol. You'll find the herb in many throat sprays, cough syrups, and lozenges. The antiseptic oil also is used in Listerine and Vick's VapoRub.

Taking thyme: To make thyme tea, steep 1 teaspoon dried thyme (or 1 tablespoon fresh) in 1 cup of water for 10 minutes; strain and drink up to three cups daily.

Safety concerns: In medicinal doses, do not give thyme

Baked Tilapia with Thyme

Ingredients
- Extra virgin olive oil
- 1 onion, chopped
- 2 lemons, halved and thinly sliced
- 1 cup green olives, halved
- 8 to 10 thyme sprigs
- Four 6-ounce tilapia fillets
- Salt
- Freshly ground pepper
- Fresh thyme sprigs, for garnish

Directions: Preheat oven to 375 F. Coat a 15- by 10- by 1-inch baking pan with olive oil. Place onion, lemon slices, olives, and thyme in bottom of pan; top with tilapia fillets. Sprinkle lightly with salt and pepper. Drizzle with olive oil.

Bake 12 to 15 minutes, or until fish flakes with a fork.

Serve immediately. Garnish each serving with a sprig of thyme. **Serves 4.**

Recipe courtesy Caleb Melchior, a freelancer from Kirkwood, Missouri.

to children younger than 2 years old. Pregnant women should not use the herb in medicinal amounts.

Fenugreek for Blood Sugar, Cholesterol, and More

With a flavor often described as similar to maple syrup, ground fenugreek seeds are a key ingredient in curry powders and other spice blends. The herb has a long history of use by nursing mothers to increase breast milk production. A 1996 study conducted in India showed that fenugreek can help lower blood sugar and cholesterol levels in type 2 diabetics. The research subjects were instructed to make no dietary or lifestyle changes, only to eat a bowl of soup that contained almost an ounce (25 grams) of fenugreek seed powder before each meal. After 24 weeks, cholesterol and blood sugar levels fell significantly.

Taking fenugreek: Make a tea by simmering 1 to 2 tablespoons fenugreek seeds in 4 cups of water for 15 minutes; remove from heat and let steep another 15 minutes, then strain and drink up to three cups daily.

Safety concerns: Avoid fenugreek during pregnancy. 🌿

Amy Mayfield was the copy editor for *Mother Earth Living*. She lives in Corvallis, Oregon, with her family.

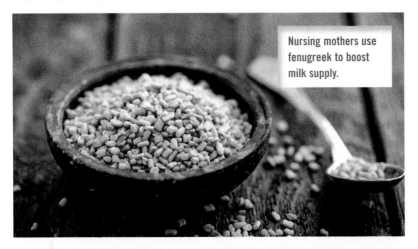

Nursing mothers use fenugreek to boost milk supply.

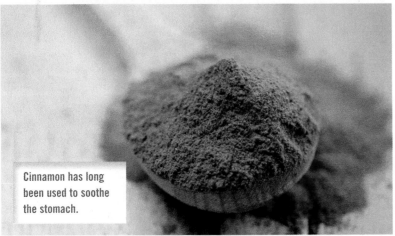

Cinnamon has long been used to soothe the stomach.

Spicy Tomato-Olive Soup

This soup is simple to make and pleasing served hot or cold. It's best if made with flavorful olive oil and high-quality olives such as Kalamata. **Serves 4 to 6.**

Ingredients
- 2 tablespoons extra virgin olive oil
- 4 large cloves garlic, crushed
- 1 large onion, coarsely chopped
- 2 tablespoons flour
- 4 cups chopped fresh tomatoes, or one 32-ounce can chopped tomatoes
- 2 cups water
- 1 teaspoon fresh or dried thyme leaves, or ¼ cup chopped fresh parsley, or 2 tablespoons minced celery leaves
- ¼ teaspoon freshly ground black pepper
- 1 to 2 tablespoons sugar, divided
- ¼ cup minced olives
- 1½ teaspoons turmeric
- Tabasco or similar hot sauce (optional)
- Salt, to taste

Directions: Heat oil in a stock pot over a moderate flame and sauté garlic until fragrant.

Stir in onion. Cook until limp, then sprinkle flour over garlic and onion. Stir and cook for 1 minute over medium heat. Add a few tablespoons of tomatoes to stock pot and stir until flour forms a smooth paste. Then slowly stir in remaining tomatoes, water, herbs, pepper, and half the sugar.

Cover and simmer 20 minutes if using canned tomatoes, 30 minutes if using fresh.

Transfer mixture to a blender and purée. Pour it back into the pot. Stir in olives and turmeric, then add additional sugar, hot sauce, and salt to taste.

Heat until very hot, then serve. It can also be chilled and served cold.

Recipe courtesy Cornelia Carlson, the author of The Practically Meatless *Gourmet.*

Plant Your *Medicine*

Grow your own healing garden with these six easy-to-grow, tasty, medicinal herbs.

By *Mother Earth News* editors

Humble though it may seem, an herb garden is truly a wonder of nature. Many herbs offer compounds known to ward off ailments and illnesses ranging from memory loss to stiff joints. Using culinary herbs to flavor food can also improve the healthfulness of our diets by helping us reduce our intake of fats and salts, instead flavoring dishes with the bright taste of homegrown herbs. And growing an herb garden offers a huge bang for your buck, as fresh culinary herbs are often expensive to buy but cheap to grow. All the herbs listed here are easy to grow, yummy to eat or drink, and offer medicinal value. Plant our six picks for a garden of good health.

Note: Herbs grown in pots indoors like frequent applications of organic fertilizer. Alternatively, simply grow these potted herbs for a few months, then replace them with new plants when their health begins to wane.

German Chamomile

Chamomile (*Matricaria chamomilla*) is reputed to help reduce anxiety and bring on sleep, both of which are crucial to our health. Argentinean researchers discovered that a compound in chamomile oil binds to the same receptors as the Valium family of tranquilizers and anti-anxiety drugs. When Japanese researchers exposed animals under stress to chamomile vapors, the animals' stress-hormone levels fell significantly. Chamomile can also soothe upset stomachs and relieve menstrual cramps.

Grow It: This annual bushy shrub is easy to grow from seed or from cutting. It's extremely low-maintenance outdoors in full sun, and you can also grow potted chamomile indoors provided you have a very sunny window or place it under fluorescent or grow lights. Chamomile requires lots of room, so plant it in a 12-inch pot in sandy, well-drained soil.

Drink It: To make a tea, pick chamomile flowers and lay them out to dry at room temperature out of direct sun for about a week. Store in a dry, well-sealed jar. Steep 1 to 2 tablespoons of dried blossoms in boiling water for about 10 minutes.

Oregano

Studies have found a compound in oregano called carvacrol to help prevent inflammation, which may help it protect against arthritis. Oregano is also high in several antioxidants including phenols and flavonoids, both of which are thought to protect against chronic diseases such as cancer.

Grow It: Hardy, perennial oregano is extremely easy to grow provided it has ample light. Find a window with at least six hours of bright light, or place oregano under fluorescent or grow lights. Grow oregano in 6-inch pots and it will assume a trailing nature.

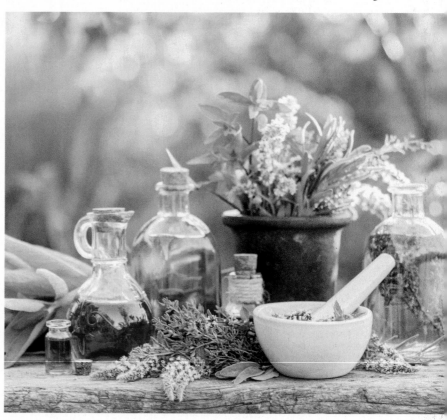

Pinch off leaves regularly to encourage an increased harvest. Plant in well-draining soil, and let soil dry slightly between waterings.

Eat It: A classic in Italian sauces such as marinara and pizza sauce, oregano is also extremely common in both Mediterranean and Mexican cooking. Add oregano to poultry, seafood, chili, vinaigrettes, and more.

Peppermint

Peppermint is a potent stomach-soother; studies have found it to relieve digestive distress in sufferers of chronic indigestion. A mild anesthetic, peppermint can also help ease the pain of sore throats. Menthol, its active ingredient, helps treat colds and congestion.

Grow It: Peppermint is among the hardiest plants in the garden. It can grow in partial sun and will grow well indoors from seed provided it gets at least some sun each day. Peppermint doesn't need much water; allow soil to dry between waterings. Peppermint needs room to spread. Plant seeds in a large pot, then thin to one plant every 12 inches once plants reach about 2 inches tall. Even one strong seedling will quickly spread to fill an entire pot.

Eat It: Peppermint makes a delicious hot or iced tea, and can also be muddled and mixed with soda water (and sugar, if desired) for a refreshing beverage. Mint is common in Thai dishes such as spring rolls and Middle Eastern dishes such as tabbouleh salad. You can also make a simple mint sauce to complement lamb or other meats by combining fresh mint with sugar and vinegar.

Rosemary

Known as the "herb of remembrance," noted herbalist James Duke says rosemary contains more than a dozen antioxidants that slow the breakdown of acetylcholine, a neurotransmitter that aids in memory and may help ward off Alzheimer's disease.

Grow It: Drainage and light are both crucial for rosemary. Line rosemary pots with 1½ to 2 inches of gravel or perlite below a fast-draining

soil mix. Place pots on a saucer, then water from the bottom by filling the tray with water. Rosemary needs lots of light, so place it in a west- or south-facing sunny window or under fluorescent lights. Moving air will help prevent powdery mildew, which often plagues indoor rosemary. Ventilate plants with a small fan. If you see rosemary leaves going white with mildew, snip off the affected areas, then spray the plant with a mixture of 2 tablespoons milk per cup of water.

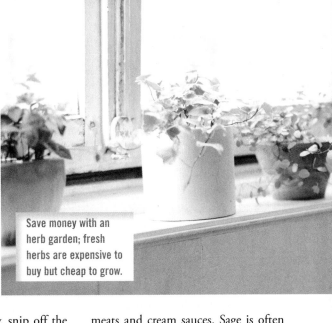

Save money with an herb garden; fresh herbs are expensive to buy but cheap to grow.

Eat It: A classic flavoring for roast chicken, rosemary works well with almost any poultry, beef, pork, or fish recipe, as well as on potatoes or in flatbread.

Sage

Sage has multiple health benefits. It's been found to enhance memory, particularly in the elderly. Sage is an excellent source of vitamin K and is rich in numerous antioxidants. A 2010 study published in the *Journal of Medicinal Food* found sage particularly effective against oxidative stress in liver cells. Studies have also found sage to be a potent antibacterial, adept at killing common pathogens such as salmonella and staphylococcus.

Grow It: A Mediterranean native, sage is an extremely hardy perennial and will survive winters outdoors in most climates. It requires lots of sun and excellent drainage, so make sure not to overwater. If growing sage indoors, include a 1½- to 2-inch layer of gravel or perlite below well-drained potting mix. Sage needs lots of sun, so unless you have a sun room, consider using a grow light or fluorescent lights placed 6 inches above the plant and left on for 14 hours a day.

Eat It: Sage's robust flavor holds up to strong, rich ingredients such as

meats and cream sauces. Sage is often used in sausages, stuffings, cream pasta sauces, and baked goods such as cornbread. You can also brew a tasty tea by steeping fresh leaves in boiling water.

Thyme

In Europe, health-care practitioners use a variety of thyme products to treat coughs, bronchitis, emphysema, and even asthma. The German Commission E (a German governmental health regulatory agency) considers thyme a bronchospasmolytic, expectorant, and antibacterial. In a German study including more than 7,000 patients, a treatment of dried primula root and thyme extract proved as effective as synthetic drugs in treating bronchitis.

Grow It: Although you can propagate thyme easily from cuttings or plant divisions, you can also purchase small thyme plants and keep them alive on a windowsill while you eat them, then buy a new plant. Thyme prefers full sun, so grow it in a sunny window or under fluorescent or grow lights. Drought-resistant thyme needs infrequent watering and well-drained soil.

Eat It: Thyme commonly flavors soups, stocks, and stews. It is a crucial element in many French and Middle Eastern dishes, including the classic French flavoring herbes de Provence. In the Middle East, it is combined with oregano and marjoram in the spice blend za'atar, used in flatbreads and to flavor meats. ❧

Houseplants for *Herbalists*

Get the most enjoyment and utility out of your houseplants by growing those that double as medicinal sources.

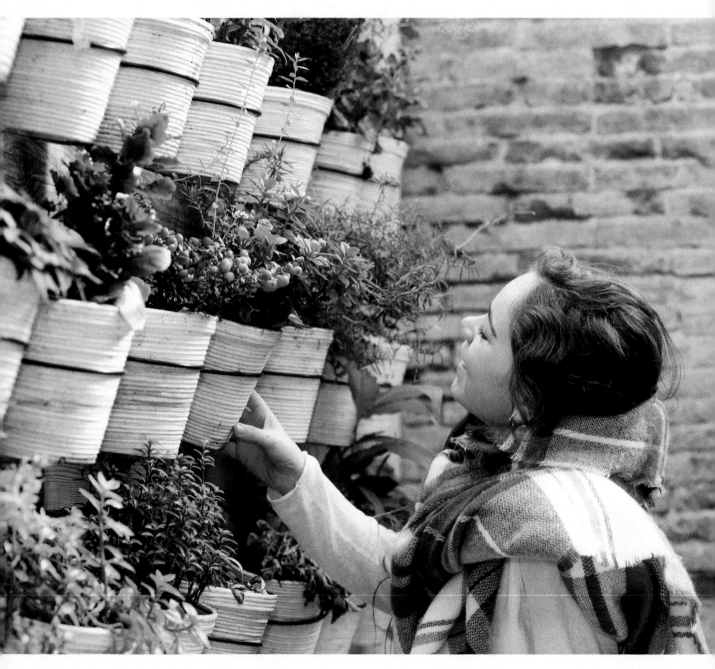

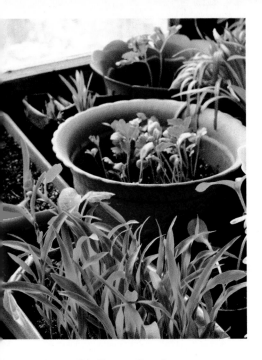

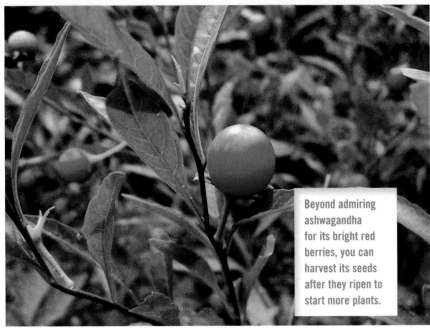

Beyond admiring ashwagandha for its bright red berries, you can harvest its seeds after they ripen to start more plants.

By Dawn Combs

Most of us have the philosophy that it's better to buy fruit from the farmer down the road—or pick it out of our backyard—than get it from the grocery store, especially if it has spent a week in transit from the other side of the planet. We still struggle, however, with the idea that our medicines should be given the same consideration. Most medicinal plants are at their best just after you harvest them, giving you the highest nutrient levels and medicinal compounds when used fresh. Local medicine is the basis of my book *Heal Local*, and it has become my mission to spread the word that your astragalus root should be just as fresh and local as your carrots.

The idea of local medicine is understandable when we apply it to parsley and peppermint, which are readily available during the growing season at most farmers markets. But what about when our medicine of choice is a tropical plant and we live in a temperate zone? This gap is a perfect space for creativity in our choice of houseplants.

For years, I've experimented with growing the herbs we need for our family both on our land and in pots. Some of my houseplants live in the ground during the summer months and then "fly south" for the winter to a sunny, indoor windowsill. Keep in mind that if you would like to try growing your medicinals in pots, you will need to research their individual needs. If you don't understand the environment where they grow naturally in the ground, you won't be able to mimic that in the pot.

Listed here are a few of my favorites, or rather, the ones I haven't killed! I'm afraid I'm a bit of an indoor plant failure. Take it from me—if I've had success with the following oddities, you can as well.

When planning to use any new herb as a food or medicinal source, consult your health-care practitioner in order to pinpoint any potential contraindications with existing medications, and take precautions when ingesting a new herb for the first time.

Gotu Kola (*Centella asiatica*)

Gotu kola is native to India. It grows in ditches and wet areas, forming a creeping mat of shiny, green leaves. Gotu kola has a place in both Chinese and Ayurvedic medicinal practices and a long history of use given the benefits it bestows on our cognitive abilities.

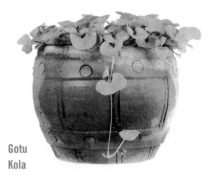

Gotu Kola

How to use: Gotu kola leaves are delicious! They can be simple grazing snacks, and you can add them to salads, smoothies, pestos, sauces, and more. The leaves are traditionally infused into teas and oils but are typically not heated so as to protect their delicate phytochemicals.

How to start: Gotu kola isn't a great option for starting as a seed unless you are very patient. You'll do better buying a plant or taking a cutting from someone you know.

How to grow: I grow my gotu kola in a wide pot, as it likes room to ramble. You might even want to hang it to allow the escaping tendrils to dangle. Gotu kola shouldn't dry out, so don't make or buy a potting mix that is filled with too much perlite or sand. My kitchen is a great place to keep gotu kola because there are a number of spots where I can keep the pot out of direct sunlight; it likes to be shaded, so keep it in a warm area away from any windows. Depending on whether your house is situated in a humid or arid environment, you may need to mist the plant often in addition to keeping it evenly watered.

Ashwagandha (*Withania somnifera*)

Ashwagandha is a pretty little plant with green leaves and red berries that is native to the dry parts of India. It's in the same family as the pepper, eggplant, and tomato (Solanaceae or nightshade), so it's no surprise ashwagandha resembles the latter fruit. This is one of my indoor/outdoor houseplants. I always move it outside when the weather gets reliably warm in the spring and then bring it back inside in the fall.

How to use: Throughout the growing season, you can pick off the leaves of a healthy ashwagandha plant and use them in teas. If you carefully dig around the outside edges of your pot, you will find roots that are harvestable. Wait to cut these roots until after the berries have ripened. With a sharp, clean knife, harvest small roots, and then carefully bury the plant again in moist soil. Medicinally, ashwagandha is used as an adaptogen, supporting the immune system and the endocrine system, and reducing stress. You can let the berries ripen and save seeds to start more plants.

How to start: Ashwagandha is not difficult to start from seed. It's a light-dependent germinator, so sow it along the top of the soil, water well, and cover with plastic. Ashwagandha is a relatively easy plant to find, so if you want to start from the very beginning by planting it yourself, then you should have no trouble.

How to grow: Ashwagandha doesn't like wet feet. The best soil mix for this plant has a high concentration of sand or drainage materials. Ashwagandha should only be watered when the soil dries out. If you're keeping it inside year-

round, you'll need a sunny spot that's fairly warm, somewhere between 70 and 85 degrees. If it's a winter-only houseplant, my recommendation is to place it in a spot that's 50 to 60 degrees so it remains healthy.

Lemongrass (*Cymbopogon citratus*)

I never liked the already dried lemongrass I bought from herb companies. When I grew my own outdoors, however, I quickly realized fresh is best. I love having this aromatic and useful plant around throughout the season. This year, I'm growing my supply in the house so I never have to go without the delicious, uplifting smell of fresh-cut lemongrass.

How to use: If you're planning to use your lemongrass plant for cooking, you'll most likely use the bulb and grass. For medicinal purposes, you only need the stalk. This herb can be turned into a number of medicinal preparations, but to me the most delightful use is in a tea. The name says it all: Lemongrass gives your drink a pleasant lemon flavor. As mild as it seems compared to other herbal tastes, it has quite a long list of purported benefits. Though studies are still preliminary in some areas, a collection of them have shown lemongrass can help alleviate nausea, support the digestive system, maintain good cholesterol, relax the nervous system, and more. Mix lemongrass into warm tea or bathwater.

How to start: Lemongrass is available for purchase in many grocery stores these days. What you buy as produce is actually a part of the grass stalk with the bulb below. In this state, it's so easy to replant. After you cut off the grass that you need for your recipe, place the bulb directly in moist soil and allow it to root. Leave only about 2 inches of grass

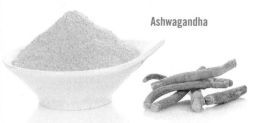

Ashwagandha

Houseplant Seed Source

Are you looking to start your herbal houseplant collection? For seeds, we recommend Strictly Medicinal Seeds (StrictlyMedicinalSeeds.com). Founded by Richo Cech, author of *Making Plant Medicine*, Strictly Medicinal provides seeds and starts for a number of unique medicinal plants that are difficult to find elsewhere. You can find seeds for all of the plants mentioned in this article, and many more, in their extensive catalogs.

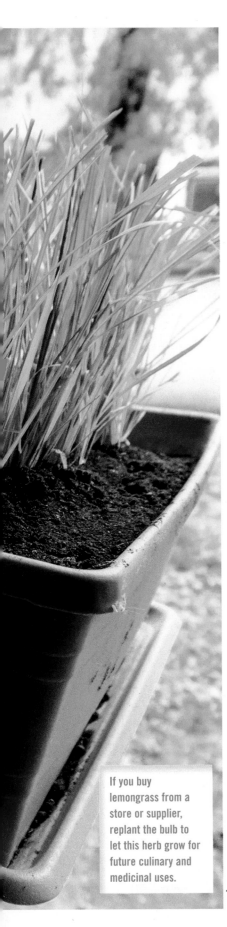

If you buy lemongrass from a store or supplier, replant the bulb to let this herb grow for future culinary and medicinal uses.

above the bulb or the plant will be too dried out and stressed to survive. Plants are also available from many suppliers, if you wish to go that route.

How to grow: Lemongrass likes full sun and moist but well-drained soil. You need to think ahead when choosing a pot for this plant, as it likes to spread. In fact, the more you harvest, the more you stimulate it to grow. A little tip: Set this plant out of your cat's reach because it might be disappointing when they've slobbered all over what you were planning to harvest for dinner.

Passionflower (*Passiflora incarnata*)

I don't really need to grow this plant indoors because it's hardy in my part of the country, Zone 6a. Of course, being hardy only means my passionflower vine will live through the winter and reemerge in the spring, not that it will remain green and useful across all seasons. If I want to continue to harvest the fresh leaves when the snow falls, I have to have one growing inside. My favorite part of the house for a passionflower vine is in the alcove with my large garden bathtub. In the summer months, when the otherworldly purple blooms appear, it's an amazing place to soak and relax.

How to use: The leaf of passionflower is a nervine and a sedative, providing relief for many who struggle with insomnia, stress, and anxiety. It has also been shown to help lower blood pressure. Typically passionflower is used internally, so leaves can be made into teas or tinctures right off the plant throughout the year. This vine likes to be pruned, so the more you use it, the better it will grow.

How to start: Passionflower can be slow to germinate, so most people buy plants or take cuttings from a friend.

How to grow: Passionflower is a vine. It's hardy in Zones 7 to 10 and

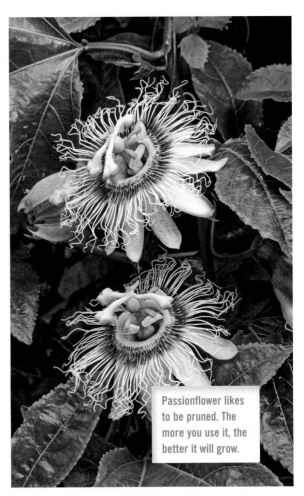

Passionflower likes to be pruned. The more you use it, the better it will grow.

will die back to the ground only to return after the winter in temperate areas. Indoors, the plant likes well-drained soil. During spring, summer, and fall, it likes to be watered on a routine basis; during winter you can let it dry out between waterings. Place it in a spot that gets full sun and stays between 65 and 85 degrees.

No matter how you choose to use these plants, they provide both beauty and benefits. From my practical point of view, if you're going to provide a space for them and spend energy keeping them alive, why not grow houseplants that are also useful? 🌿

Dawn Combs is the author of *Heal Local* and the co-owner of Mockingbird Meadows Herbal Health Farm, where she provides on-site education about herbs. Find Dawn at Mocking BirdMeadows.com.

A GUIDE TO
Drying Herbs

Growing and drying herbs and spices is among
the easiest forms of food preservation.

By Tabitha Alterman

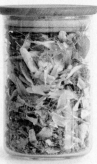

W hen it comes to preserving our own food, growing and drying herbs is one of the best jumping-off points. Many herbs are incredibly easy to grow, and most contain so little moisture that the preservation job is done soon after they're harvested. Drying herbs and spices also makes good economic sense considering the cost of high-quality seasonings and teas. And when we grow our own, we know with certainty we are getting herbs that are both fresh and organic. Lastly, when you grow your own herbs, you can grow the particular varieties that appeal to you and experiment with creating your own custom herb blends.

Herb and Spice Drying Basics

According to *The Deluxe Food Lover's Companion* by Sharon Tyler Herbst and Ron Herbst, culinary herbs are leaves, while spices are obtained from the bark, berries, buds

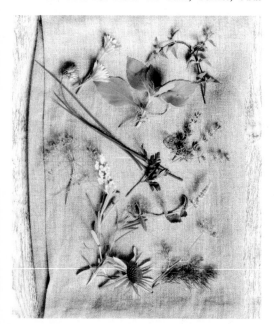

(and even flower stigmas), fruit, roots, and seeds of plants. Spices are almost always used in dried form, whereas herbs can be used fresh or dried. Here are a few examples: bark (cinnamon); berries (peppercorns); buds (cloves, lavender); fruit (chili peppers, vanilla beans); leaf (cilantro, parsley); roots (garlic, horseradish); seeds (coriander, juniper); and stigma (saffron).

To preserve your homegrown herbs, harvest them in midmorning before newly developed essential oils have been burned off by the sun, but after the dew has dried. Remove old, dead, diseased, or wilted leaves. Washing fresh herbs usually isn't necessary if they are grown organically.

When you harvest seed spices, the seed heads should begin to turn brown and harden, but not yet be ready to shatter. To harvest herbs for their flowers—such as chamomile flowers or thyme spikes— snip flower buds off the plants close to the first day the buds open.

Fully dried herbs and spices are safe from bacteria, mold, and yeast, and will remain potent for at least six to 12 months. To remove moisture, all you need is air circulation. Some warmth can also help. The six methods detailed here fit the bill.

Indoor Air-Drying: To air-dry herbs on stems, tie stems in bundles and hang the herbs upside down in a warm, dry place (avoid the kitchen, a source of steam and cooking vapors). Use twist-ties or thin-gauge wire so you can easily tighten the bundles as the drying stems shrink. Wrap bundles with muslin, a mesh produce bag, or a paper bag with several holes, and tie it at the neck. If you're drying individual leaves, flowers, or sprigs, make a drying screen from an old window screen or hardware cloth or mesh stapled to a wooden frame. Lay cheesecloth over the screen, and place herbs on the cloth.

Storing Dried Herbs & Spices

Herbs and spices have finished drying when the leaves crumble easily and no longer feel leathery; don't crumble them. Whole leaves and seeds retain their oils better in storage. Store dried herbs in airtight jars out of direct light and away from heat. Label jars immediately with the date and contents, including the specific variety so you can pinpoint favorites. After a few days, check new jars for droplets of moisture or mold. Throw out anything moldy; redry anything that creates moisture in the jar.

Although whole herbs and spices hold up better, having premixed ground blends—such as those for Italian, Mexican, or barbecue dishes—can be a timesaver (to make an Italian herb blend, mix 2½ tablespoons each dried oregano and basil and 1 generous tablespoon dried marjoram). Grind ingredients with a mortar and pestle. When using dried herbs in recipes that call for fresh, remember that oils in dried herbs are more concentrated. Use half the amount of dried herbs, and a quarter as much if the herb is finely ground.

Tea blends are also useful, such as peppermint and fennel to calm an upset stomach. To use herbs in teas, pour boiling water over a teaspoon to a tablespoon (to taste) of the dried herb and steep for 5 to 10 minutes. Strain and enjoy.

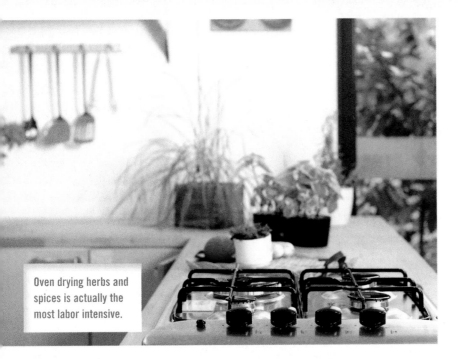

Oven drying herbs and spices is actually the most labor intensive.

Once herbs are fully dry, which can take anywhere from a few hours to a few days, prepare them for storage as outlined in "Storing Dried Herbs & Spices" on page 46.

Solar Drying: This method is ideal for warm, dry weather around 100 degrees and 60 percent humidity or less. In these conditions, you can use the sun's heat to dry herbs. Don't expose herbs to too much direct sunlight as this could cause them to bleach. Solar drying can be as low-tech as placing drying screens outside until your herbs are brittle (bring them in at night). You can also dry herbs under the windshield or rear window of your car on a hot day. Or build your own solar food dehydrator with stackable drying screens, a glass top to trap radiation, an absorber plate to transmit heat, and a vent for air circulation. Find building plans online at MotherEarthNews.com/Herb-Drying-Guide.

Refrigerator Drying: Another super-simple method of drying herbs basically amounts to neglect. Just stick them in the fridge and forget about them for a few days. This handy tip was discovered by the late herb authority Madalene Hill and her daughter Gwen Barclay. By accident, they discovered that herbs left alone (out of packaging) in a cold, dry refrigerator dried beautifully crisp and also retained their color, flavor, and fragrance. They even liked this method for parsley and chives, which don't have the best reputation for keeping great flavor in dried form. The challenge is finding enough room to let herbs sit uncovered for a few days. If your fridge has available space, by all means, give it a try.

Dehydrating With a Machine: Commercial food dehydrators range in price from $30 to $400, but for most of us, a machine that costs $100 to $200 is the best choice. Quality dehydrators have handy features such as timers and adjustable temperature control. Stored in a convenient spot, you'll use your dehydrator often and recoup its cost in a season or two of grocery savings.

Most dehydrators have a temperature-control mechanism—ideally one you can adjust—and a fan to circulate air. Round models with multiple stacking trays are the most energy-efficient. Box-type models that allow you to remove some of the trays can be handy for drying large items and can serve other purposes such as proofing bread dough or culturing yogurt. Follow your machine's instructions.

Oven Drying: Although drying herbs and spices in an oven sounds easy (most of us already have one and know how to use it), this is actually the most labor-intensive and least energy-efficient method. Herbs need to be dried at about 100 degrees, but most ovens don't go that low. They also need air circulation, and some ovens don't have vents. If you wish to dry your herbs this way, it's best to get an oven thermometer and experiment. Try turning the oven on warm or its lowest setting for a while, then turning it off (while leaving the light on). You can also try propping the door open slightly with a wooden spoon. Note how long it takes for the temperature to drop to 100 degrees and how long it stays at that temperature.

Herbs are far easier than fruits and vegetables to oven-dry because they dry more quickly and are more forgiving. If you plan to learn how to use your oven for food dehydration, definitely start with herbs. Layer them on a cheesecloth over a wire cooling rack to allow for air circulation all around, and place the rack in the middle of the oven when the temperature is about 100 degrees.

Microwave Drying: The microwave can successfully dry herbs, but note that food-drying experts do not recommend it for drying foods that have more moisture. It's not as easy as air-drying or using an electric dehydrator.

To dry herbs in a microwave, strip leaves off of the stems and place the leaves between layers of paper towels. Begin on high power for 1 minute, allow a 30-second rest, and then alternate between 30 seconds on high power and 30 seconds of rest. Most herbs should dry fully in 10 minutes or less. 🌿

Tabitha Alterman was the Food & Garden editor for *Mother Earth Living*.

Freezing Herbs

Some herbs, although they can be dried, retain their flavor better if frozen. These include basil, borage, chives, cilantro, lemongrass, mint, and parsley. To freeze herbs, chop them and put them in ice cube trays, then cover with water and freeze. Alternatively, mix chopped herbs with a bit of olive oil and freeze. Use frozen herbs in dishes where they will melt easily, such as soups, sauces, and stir-fries.

BOOST
your Immunity

Get ready for fall and winter with these powerful immune boosters.

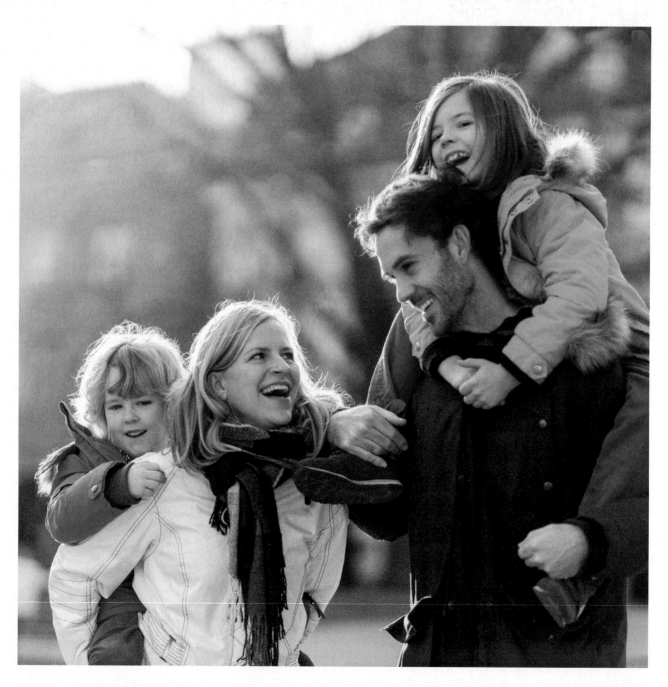

By Kris Wetherbee

The last decade alone has seen an influx of infectious diseases and virulent strains increasingly unaffected by conventional treatments. Overuse and abuse of antibiotic medicines and antibacterial products have turned the war on germs into a war on humankind as once-common bacteria and viruses mutate to new levels of resistance. According to a 1992 article in *Science*, "doctors in hospitals and clinics around the world are losing the battle against an onslaught of new drug-resistant bacterial infections and other diseases that are costly and difficult, if not impossible, to treat."

You may not be able to avoid the onslaught of bacteria, viruses, and other germs capable of wreaking havoc in your body. However, you can take the offensive by revving up your immune system so your body can more effectively resist whatever diseases come your way.

Running on Empty

Everyday life is full of encounters from any number of pathogens and foreign substances that can infiltrate and attack your body. Your immune system defends your body against these invaders. An intricate network of cells, tissues, and organs, your immune system fights back by detecting and destroying any substance that doesn't belong in your body.

But when your immune system is compromised, a breakdown occurs that can make you more susceptible to diseases and infections. Physical, psychological, and social factors ranging from sustained stress and environmental toxins to poor diet and lifestyle choices can leave your body running on empty. For example, high cholesterol and alcohol can suppress immune activity that fights infection, and sustained stress affects hormone levels that regulate immune functions. Refined sugars and excess natural sugars can weaken your immunity as well. According to a 1977 study published in the *American Journal of Clinical Nutrition*, drinking 24 ounces of sugary soda depressed infection-fighting white blood cell activity by 50 percent for about five hours after consumption.

Fortunately, nature has provided plants that can enhance and restore immune function. Scientific studies are verifying the immune-boosting and antimicrobial actions of botanical medicines and their synergistic mix of plant-based chemicals that may help prevent diseases from colds to cancer.

The Familiar Five

Herbs like echinacea (*Echinacea* spp.), Asian ginseng (*Panax ginseng*), eleuthero (*Eleutherococcus senticosus*), garlic (*Allium sativum*), and green tea (*Camellia sinensis*) have become common household names, and with good reason. They all possess elements that modulate, activate, or enhance immune function and the antimicrobial properties that fight disease.

One of the most popular is echinacea, which contains a number of antioxidant compounds and immune-stimulating constituents that can help the immune system fight off illness.

According to a University of Florida study, echinacea was

Fighting a Cold or Flu

Immune-boosting herbs are most effective when taken as preventives or at the very first sign of illness. Though prevention is preferred, there will likely be times when outside forces get the better of your immune system and you end up succumbing to the seasonal cold or flu. Herbal antibiotics like echinacea, garlic, and licorice can help you fight back. Goldenseal (*Hydrastis canadensis*) and Oregon grape (*Mahonia aquifolium*) contain phytochemical compounds, including berberine, a natural alkaloid that increases infection-fighting white blood cells.

If your medicinal cupboard is bare, you may still find relief in your herb and spice rack. The astringent and antiseptic tannins found in basil and sage are great for reducing oral inflammation. Try a warm sage tea and salt gargle to cool down the pain and inflammation of a sore throat. The menthol in peppermint and the anti-inflammatory actions of capsicum —found in cayenne—make powerful decongestants for opening up mucous membranes.

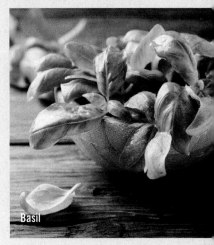

Basil

shown to stimulate threefold the activity of infection-fighting immune-system cells. Taken at the first sign of illness, the dosage can make a difference between you beating the bug or the bug beating you.

"Three to four capsules a day is inadequate when you get sick," says Majid Ali, an herbalist and acupuncturist in Santa Monica, California. When symptoms are really bad, Ali has his patients take one or two capsules (300 to 400 mg each) every hour, or two for the first 24 to 48 hours (until they feel better), then continue with one or two capsules four times daily for three to five days after symptoms disappear.

Garlic is a potent antioxidant packed with antimicrobial compounds like cancer-fighting sulfur and the immune-boosting mineral selenium. Perhaps the most beneficial compound in garlic is allicin. Heating or cooking garlic inactivates the enzyme that produces allicin, but if garlic is chopped and allowed to sit for 10 minutes before cooking, enough allicin is formed to maintain the healthful benefits. Exposing garlic to heat for as little time as possible (lightly sautéing, for example) will help retain its enzyme activity. Of course, the best way to enjoy the healthful properties of garlic is to consume one raw clove a day, but many people find raw garlic difficult to digest.

Active antioxidants also can be found in green tea, Asian ginseng, and eleuthero. In studies, green tea has shown the ability to modulate immune function. Preliminary research

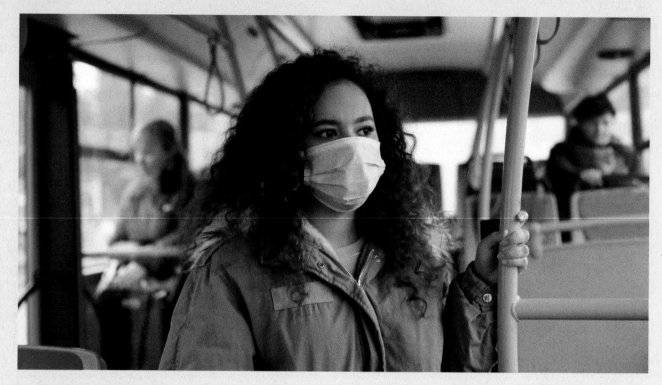

Suppressing SARS?

The following article was originally published in 2003, shortly after SARS was first reported. The illness spread to more than two dozen countries before the outbreak was contained. Since 2004, there have not been any known cases of SARS reported anywhere in the world.

Can boosting your immunity slap SARS silly? Maybe, according to James Duke, Ph.D., a 30-year veteran of the USDA and one of the world's foremost authorities on herbal medicine. Herbs haven't been shown to kill the bug responsible for Severe Acute Respiratory Syndrome, but using herbs regularly may well give our own bodies the oomph they need to fend off this and many other diseases, Duke says.

"Our public health people recommend seeing your physician or health-care professional if you suspect you might have SARS," he says. "But they confess there isn't much they can do but provide supportive treatment. They all say contagious diseases are more likely to gain a foothold in, infect, and even kill those with compromised immune systems.

"It simply stands to reason that the corollary is that a strong immune system renders the acquisition of most contagious diseases —among them anthrax, SARS, smallpox, and West Nile virus—less likely. Strengthening the immune system can be preventive."

Duke suggests lifestyle changes to boost the immune system, including:

- Eat a diet featuring lots of fresh fruits and vegetables (nine servings a day).
- Take a daily multivitamin.
- Relax and reduce stress.
- Think positive.
- Exercise, but don't overdo it. Take in some fresh air every day—walk in the garden, stroll around your neighborhood, sit on a park bench—just make sure you breathe deeply.
- Take herbs reported to boost immunity when contagious diseases are going around.

Garlic leads the list of herbs Duke recommends because it contains at least 15 immune-boosting chemicals, 10 antiviral agents, and at least 24 antibacterial compounds. It has been proven synergistic with many of the pharmaceutical antibiotics, which are losing their punch due to multiple drug resistance.

Try the whole garlic, not the "deodorized" version, Duke says. "The more it stinks, the better its success as an antiseptic, immune booster, and mosquito repellent." (Mosquitoes carry the West Nile virus.)

Green tea also is high on the list of herbs Duke recommends.

"Experiments show that immune system blood cells of tea drinkers responded five times more rapidly to germs than did the blood cells of coffee drinkers," he says. "The process by which the liver breaks down tea prompts the secretion of interferon, an important part of the body's chemical defense against infection."

Concerned about contagion? Here's Duke's advice: "I'd prop up my feet on a foot stool and drink green tea with cinnamon, ginger, and vanilla, while avoiding the depressing TV news that might counteract the immune-boosting propensities of my herbal concoction," he says.

Even if the echinacea and garlic you take as preventives enhance your immune system by only 1 or 10 percent, Duke says, that at least improves your chances of resisting disease.

"I'll take that chance over doing nothing, or passively hoping my qualified health-care professional can see me in time and has the silver bullet that will make me well," he says.

K.C. Compton

suggests that the amino acid L-theanine works to boost the capacity of specific T cells that act as the body's first line of defense against infection. Asian ginseng improved immune response according to one Italian study conducted at the University of Milan, and the results of a German study demonstrated a drastic increase in the number of immune cells in healthy volunteers taking eleuthero.

Powerful Plant Protectors

Although the name recognition of these botanical wonders may not be as common as the familiar five, their immune-enhancing qualities are just as significant. Elderberries (*Sambucus nigra*) contain anthocyanins, a group of antioxidants that increase the production of cytokines, which help protect the body against disease. Studies published in the *Journal of Alternative and Complementary Medicine* also suggest that elderberries actually can prevent a number of viral strains from replicating.

Ashwaganda (*Withania somnifera*), an Ayurvedic herb also known as Indian ginseng, is said to have adaptogenic properties that improve the body's ability to withstand adverse conditions while normalizing its immunity functions. Several animal studies conducted in India on the immune-boosting effects of ashwaganda have shown a significant increase in white blood cell counts and platelet counts.

Schisandra (*Schisandra chinensis*) acts as an adaptogen as well, according to Earl Mindell, Ph.D., author of *Prescription Alternatives*. "Schisandra has a stimulating effect on the central nervous system without causing heart palpitations or anxiety," Mindell says.

Rhodiola (*Rhodiola rosea*), also known as arctic root, is yet another adaptogenic herb that restores normal functioning of the immune system. "Almost everyone in the country could be helped with this herb, as adrenal exhaustion is so common, especially if you consume caffeine," Mindell explains. "It helps the body cope with stress, which I think is one of the biggest problems Americans face."

Astragalus (*Astragalus membranaceus*) not only functions as an adaptogen, it also stimulates natural killer cells and elevates interferon, a protein that prevents viruses from replicating. The outcome of one study (published in *World Science*) involving 1,000 people with lowered immunity resulted in fewer colds and reduced symptoms after taking astragalus. Astragalus also holds promise as an anti-cancer agent. Researchers at the University of Texas Medical Center in Houston were able to completely restore the function of cancer patients' damaged immune cells using astragalus extracts in an in vitro study.

Biological Defenders

Studies involving the immune-activating properties of fungi may still be in their infancy, but specialty mushrooms have been used in Asian medicine for more than 2,000 years.

Medicinal mushrooms are rich sources of the active anti-cancer agent beta-glucan, a polysaccharide that activates immune cells

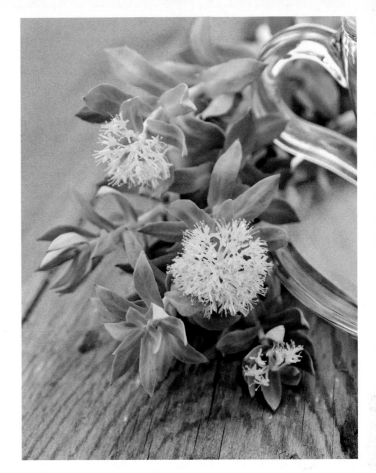

Rhodiola helps the body cope with stress.

and increases antibodies that regulate the development of defense responses. Reishi mushroom (*Ganoderma lucidum*) is a noted antioxidant that has demonstrated antibacterial effects against strep and the bacteria that lead to pneumonia. Cordyceps is another immune-modulating medicinal mushroom that possesses anti-tumor properties and stimulates tumor necrosis factor, a cytokine protein that destroys cancer cells.

Usnea (*Usnea* spp.), a lichen born from a symbiotic union between fungi and algae, is a powerful immune stimulator. A study published in the *Romanian Journal of Physiology* found its broad-spectrum antibiotic activity to be more effective than penicillin against certain bacteria, without destroying the good bacteria normally found in the intestines. Its mucilage action also helps shrink swollen mucous membranes and is great for soothing sore throats.

Food Fortification

Let's face it: Vital nutrients necessary for maintaining a healthy immune system are sorely lacking, perhaps even nonexistent, in the high-fat and sugar-laden highly processed food culture of today. Combined with the onslaught of chemical residues and added foreign substances, it would seem that the average diet is starving for essential vitamins and minerals needed for proper immunity.

In *Beyond Antibiotics*, author Michael Schmidt writes, "There is growing evidence that vitamin and mineral deficiency can lead to diminished immunity and increased infection susceptibility." Seeking out food sources rich in immune-boosting nutrients—

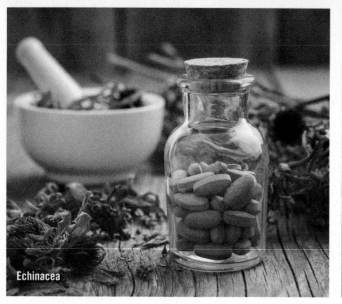
Echinacea

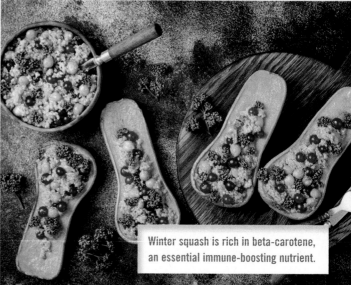
Winter squash is rich in beta-carotene, an essential immune-boosting nutrient.

such as beta-carotene, vitamin C, vitamin E, lutein, lycopene, selenium, and zinc—can help prevent nutrient deficiencies.

Many vegetables and fruits are rich in beta-carotene, especially sweet potatoes, carrots, winter squash, broccoli, cantaloupe, and apricots. Vitamin C functions as an antibacterial and antiviral player, and powerhouse sources of this nutrient include oranges, sweet peppers, strawberries, and kiwis. Vitamin E is a well-known antioxidant that also takes part in regulating immune function. Whole grains, nuts, and seeds are some of the richest sources.

Selenium-rich foods include seafood, whole grains, organ meats, garlic, and onions.

Zinc helps boost immune response, and foods like turkey, lean lamb and beef, liver, and pumpkin seeds can boost levels of zinc, a mineral USDA studies have shown is lacking in the diets of 83 percent of American women.

Antioxidant-rich carotenoids such as lycopene and lutein may help enhance immune response and protect immune cells from oxidative damage. Some of the highest food sources for lycopene include tomatoes, red grapefruit, and watermelon. Abundant sources of lutein can be found in leafy green vegetables such as spinach and kale.

A Final Word

Remember that pre-existing health conditions—from hypertension to cancer—as well as prescription medications, menopause, and pregnancy can have a direct effect on what herbs are best to take, along with when and how to take them. For example, licorice (*Glycyrrhiza glabra*) can be used as a preventive for colds and flu but would be inappropriate for someone taking high blood pressure medication.

Timing also can play a crucial part in infection prevention. "Some herbs, like echinacea, are natural antibiotics, and if taken continuously, they lose their efficacy," Ali explains. During cold and flu season, Ali advises his patients to take echinacea for just one week, followed by two weeks of astragalus and reishi. A second rotation of echinacea/astragalus is then followed by a week off of the herbs. 🌿

Kris Wetherbee is a freelance writer and was a frequent contributor to *The Herb Companion*. She lives in the hills of western Oregon with her photographer husband, Rick Wetherbee.

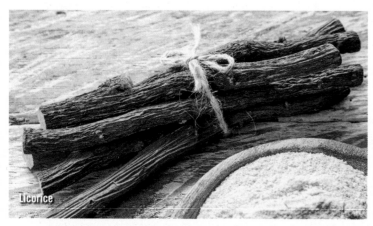
Licorice

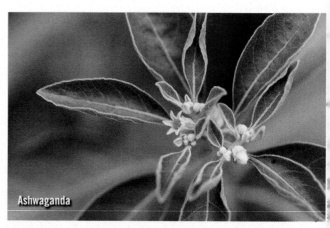
Ashwaganda

12 STRATEGIES TO STRENGTHEN YOUR IMMUNE SYSTEM

Bolster your immune system naturally with these easy tips!

By Linda B. White, M.D.

Infections are as inevitable as death and taxes. You spend your first years catching colds, influenza, and strep throat. You sniffle, scratch, cough, vomit, ache, sweat, and shiver. Your immune system remembers the microbes it has encountered and protects you the next go around. At the other end of life, your immune system wearies from years of fighting.

In that great expanse of active, productive life in between, you still get colds and flus and "stomach bugs." You may wonder why you are sick more or less often than your partner, co-workers and neighbors.

The answer is that not all immune systems function alike. A number of factors affect immune system health. Some you can't control: The very young and the very old are vulnerable. Surgery and wounds give microbes a chance to sneak into the inner sanctum. Other risks include chronic disease, poverty, stress, living with lots of other people (dormitories, low-income housing), and drinking tap water (with its local microbes) in many foreign countries. Fortunately, there are ways you can strengthen your immune system.

1. **Eat like Peter Rabbit.** Malnutrition impairs immune function. French fries, soft drinks, and bourbon don't build strong white blood cells either. Diets high in fruits, vegetables, and nuts promote immune health, presumably because they're rich in nutrients the immune system requires. Adequate protein intake is also important; the source can be plant or animal. Medicinal mushrooms such as shiitake, maitake, and reishi contain beta-glucans (complex carbohydrates) that enhance immune activity against infections and cancer, and reduce allergies (cases of inappropriate immune system activity). Although studies have focused on purified mushroom extracts, fresh

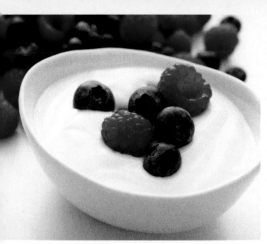
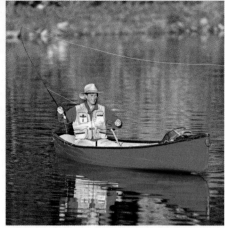

Load up on veggies, fruits, and good bacteria (yay yogurt!) to ramp up your immunity. For even better results, take time to unwind and enjoy some sun.

shiitake and maitake (also called "hen of the woods") mushrooms are delicious sautéed in a little olive oil.

One substance to avoid is simple sugar. Brigitte Mars, herbalist and author of *The Desktop Guide to Herbal Medicine*s, notes that sugary foods and juices impair immune function; research bears her out.

If you're a new mother, breast milk provides essential nutrients and immune system components to your developing child. Compared with formula-fed babies, those nourished at the breast have fewer serious infections.

2. Stress less. When you're stressed, your adrenal glands churn out epinephrine (aka adrenaline) and cortisol. While acute stress pumps up the immune system, grinding long-term duress taxes it. For instance, psychological stress raises the risk for the common cold and other viruses. Less often, chronic stress can promote a hyper-reactive immune system and aggravate conditions such as allergies, asthma, and autoimmune disease.

Although most of us can't move into a spa, we can learn to save our stress responses for true emergencies and not fire them up over stalled traffic or bad hair days. Stress-reducing activities such as meditation produce positive changes in the immune system. Massage has shown to improve immune function in studies of Dominican children with HIV. Quiet music can aid recovery from everyday hassles and may therefore buttress immune function.

3. Move your body. Moderate exercise discharges tension and stress, and enhances immune function. In a 2006 study,

researchers took 115 obese, sedentary, postmenopausal women and assigned half of them to stretching exercises once a week and the other half to at least 45 minutes of moderate-intensity exercise five days a week. At the end of the year-long study, the stretchers had three times the rate of colds as the moderate-exercise group.

4. Sleep soundly. Sleep is a time when growth-promoting and reparative hormones knit up the raveled sleeve of daily life. Sleep deprivation activates the stress response, depresses immune function, and elevates inflammatory chemicals (which cause you to feel ill).

Chronic sleep deprivation raises the risk of the common cold. Mothers whose small children interrupt their sleep have more respiratory infections, particularly if those wee ones go to day care. In one study, after researchers inoculated volunteers' noses with cold viruses (a reward was involved), men and women who habitually slept less than seven hours a night were almost three times more likely to develop a cold than those who slept eight hours or more.

5. Socialize. People with richer social lives enjoy better health and longevity than loners do. You may think that the more people you interact with, the more chances you have for picking something up. Not so. Again, researchers blew cold viruses up people's noses and sent them into the world. Compared with the lone wolves, the social butterflies were less susceptible to developing common colds, and, if they did get sick, they had fewer symptoms for a shorter period of time.

Many of us count furred and feathered

companions as friends, and it turns out they do us a world of good. Animals such as dogs and horses get us outside exercising. Stroking an animal stirs feelings of well-being, lowers blood pressure, and—according to recent research—boosts the immune system. Researchers assigned college students to pet either a stuffed dog or a live dog. Those who petted a real dog had a significant increase in levels of salivary IgG, an antibody (immune protein) that fights infection. Those who petted the stuffed dog just felt silly.

6. Make more love. Although having lots of friends is healthy, science also shows that intimate, sexual relationships may have immune system perks. Michael Castleman, renowned health writer and publisher of GreatSexGuidance.com, writes, "A 2004 study shows that the close contact of lovemaking reduces the risk of colds." Specifically, this study found that college students who had sex once or twice a week had 30 percent more salivary IgA antibody than those who had sex infrequently.

7. Shun tobacco smoke. Tobacco smoke triggers inflammation, increases respiratory mucus, and inhibits the hairlike projections inside your nose (cilia) from clearing that mucus. Children and adults exposed to tobacco smoke are more at risk for respiratory infections, including colds, bronchitis, pneumonia, sinusitis, and middle ear infections.

8. Consume friendly bacteria. Beneficial microorganisms colonize our intestinal, lower urinary, and upper respiratory tracts. They outcompete bad "bugs" and enhance immune function. You can consume such bacteria in the form of live-cultured products such as yogurt, sauerkraut, and kimchi. Probiotic supplements, available at natural food stores, may reduce the risk of antibiotic-induced diarrhea, viral diarrhea, vaginitis, and respiratory infections.

9. Expose yourself. Vitamin D plays a number of roles in promoting normal immune function. Vitamin D deficiency correlates with asthma, cancer, several autoimmune diseases (e.g., multiple sclerosis), and susceptibility to infection (including viral respiratory infections). One study linked deficiency to a greater likelihood of carrying MRSA (methicillin-resistant *Staphylococcus aureus*) in the nose.

Unfortunately, nearly one-third of the U.S. population is vitamin D deficient. Because few foods contain much vitamin D, your best bet is to regularly spend short periods of time in the sun (without sunscreen), and to take supplements in northern climes during the colder months. Guidelines for the Recommended Daily Allowance (RDA) of vitamin D, currently set at 400 IU/day, are being revised.

10. Choose vitamin and mineral supplements wisely. Studies link deficiencies of zinc, selenium, folic acid, and vitamins A, B6, C, D, and E to reduced immune function. But scientists have yet to pinpoint exact levels of these nutrients for optimal immune function, much less whether dietary supplementation really helps the average, well-fed American. For instance, research on vitamin C for prevention and treatment of the common cold has been inconclusive. Some micronutrients, notably vitamin A, can be toxic in overdose. Excessive levels of zinc paradoxically suppress immune function. A varied, plant-based diet and a good multivitamin supplement should meet your needs.

11. Immunize yourself. Routine vaccinations have had a huge impact on reducing, and in many cases nearly eradicating, a number of infectious diseases. Most immunizations occur during childhood. Vaccinations for adults to consider include yearly influenza vaccines, tetanus boosters, the shingles vaccine for people 60 and up, and the pneumococcus vaccine for people over the age of 65. For more information, check with the Centers for Disease Control (CDC.Gov/Vaccines).

12. Familiarize yourself with immune-enhancing herbs. A long list of medicinal plants contain chemicals that enhance immune system activity, including echinacea, eleuthero (also called Siberian ginseng), ginseng (Asian and American), astragalus, garlic, and shiitake, reishi, and maitake mushrooms.

Garlic is the favorite choice of many. In addition to boosting the immune system, it's anticancer and antimicrobial against a variety of bacteria, viruses, fungi, and parasites. Key ingredients don't survive cooking, so add a clove or two of raw, minced garlic to meals just before serving.

When someone in my family sniffles, I make an immune soup based on a recipe Brigitte Mars shared with me years ago: Pretend you're making chicken soup. Sauté onions, shiitake mushrooms, and chicken, adding just enough water to keep the chicken from drying out. Remove the chicken when it's cooked and set aside. Add fresh vegetables such as carrots and celery. Cover with plenty of water. Toss in three or four astragalus roots (the pressed roots, available in natural foods stores or from online herb retailers such as MountainRoseHerbs.com and PacificBotanicals.com). Toward the end of cooking, add Italian seasonings (thyme, rosemary, oregano), which are tasty and antimicrobial, and the chopped, cooked chicken.

Before serving, add fresh, pressed garlic (one to two cloves per person) and remove the astragalus roots. 🌿

Linda B. White is a Denver-based doctor, writer, and lecturer.

The Hygiene Hypothesis

Some people respond to front-page news about microbes—bird flu, flesh-eating bacteria, pathogenic E. coli—with excessive soap, water, and hand-sanitizer use, along with avoidance of fun activities such as dining out, hugging dogs, camping, French kissing, and mud wrestling. But the science says to get a little dirty. Some exposure to "germs" will mature and strengthen your immune system.

Some experts even point to evidence that an over-sanitized environment is bad for your health, increasing the risk of allergic, autoimmune, and inflammatory conditions. The so-called Hygiene Hypothesis posits that exposure to microbes early in life flexes and shapes the immune system to do what it was designed to do, like fight off the ebola virus. Growing up in an ultra-clean

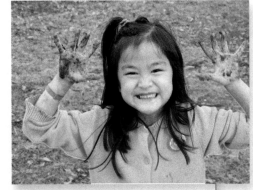

Get dirty! The Hygiene Hypothesis suggests some exposure to "germs" may be good for your health.

environment, though, may produce an immune system that attacks innocuous things (animal dander, ragweed pollen, your own cells), leading to chronic inflammation.

In support of that hypothesis, children who grow up in larger families (blessed with germy siblings), live in the country (around barnyard animals), or attend day care have lower rates of conditions such as asthma, hay fever, and eczema. On the other hand, improved sanitation (along with vaccinations and antibiotics) has clearly decreased the death rate from infections and lengthened our lives. Infections, however, continue to challenge us, which means that the Hygiene Hypothesis (and other immunity-boosting practices) is just that: a hypothesis. It remains a hot topic in immunology circles.

ISTOCK/TODDGUNKEL

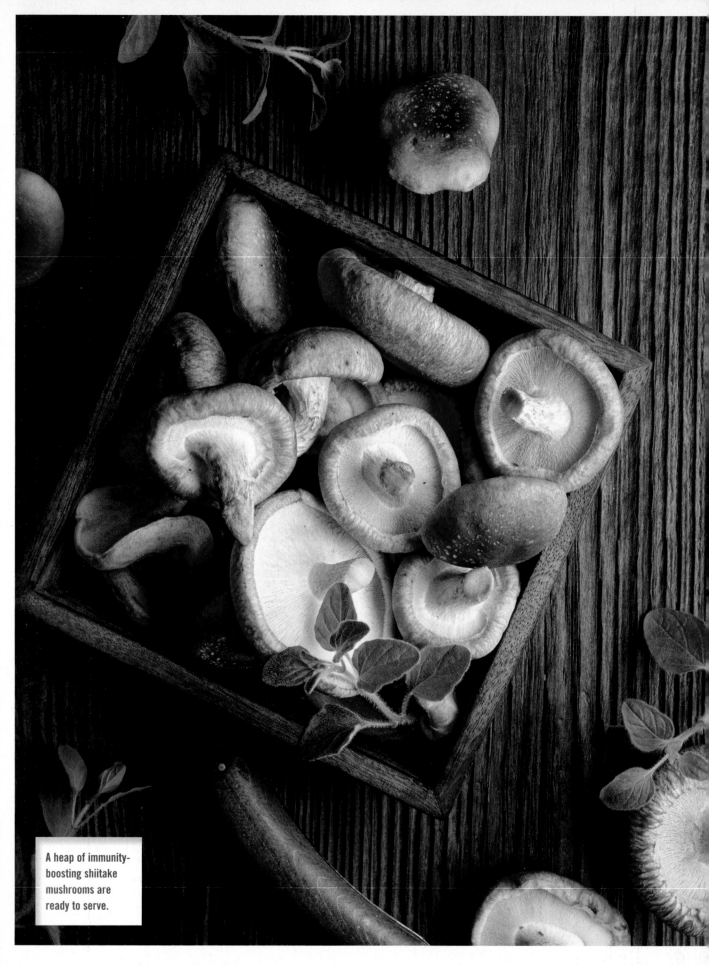

A heap of immunity-boosting shiitake mushrooms are ready to serve.

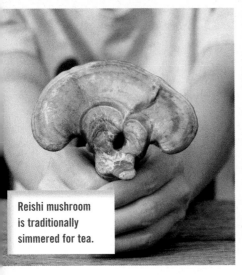

Reishi mushroom is traditionally simmered for tea.

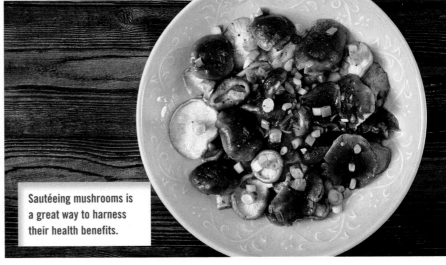

Sautéeing mushrooms is a great way to harness their health benefits.

Boost Your Immunity with Gourmet Mushrooms

Shiitake, maitake, and reishi pack potent disease-fighting compounds.

By Gina Mohammed, Ph.D.

The shiitake mushroom proves looks aren't everything: What could be scruffier or more taciturn-looking as it hunkers down on your grocer's produce shelf? Don't be so quick to judge, though. This mushroom-with-an-attitude is a study in contrasts: earthy but ethereal, unimpressive but magnificent. It performs in a cast of potent fungi known as the medicinal mushrooms, which number more than 200 worldwide and include others of sterling repute such as reishi and maitake. Unlike the Asians and Europeans who have cherished these mushrooms for millennia, we in North America are just beginning to discover their merits.

Medicinal mushrooms enhance the body's general resilience and vigor, stimulate the immune system, and confer antioxidant benefits. Since the 1960s, science has been catching up to tradition, and many clinical studies now demonstrate that these mushrooms do indeed shore up the body's defenses against such afflictions as cancer, infection, and heart disease.

Stupendous Shiitake

Our friend the shiitake (*Lentinula edodes*) is one you've probably sampled. This mushroom's meaty texture and rich, woodsy flavor make it a culinary favorite in any dish calling for mushrooms, and it is especially good in meatless cuisine. Originally from China, shiitakes have been cultivated in North America since at least the 1980s.

Shiitake protects against certain cancers, tumors, and infections—the latter through antiviral and antibiotic actions. How shiitake executes its anticancer campaign is not fully understood, but a constituent known as lentinan appears pivotal. Widely studied, lentinan from shiitake is an approved drug in Japan, used mainly as an adjunct to conventional cancer chemotherapy. Controlled clinical trials using injected lentinan with standard chemotherapy show it is effective against stomach, colorectal, and prostate cancers. In 1999, a study published in *Hepatogastroenterology* found that lentinan increased one-year survival of gastric-cancer patients to 49 percent compared to no increase without lentinan. And a trial conducted at the Saitama Cancer Center in Japan reported that five-year survival of patients with metastatic prostate cancer was 43 percent with lentinan treatment versus 29 percent without it.

Shiitake is especially rich in lentinan, a complex polysaccharide of the beta-D-glucan family found in sources such as oats, barley, yeast, algae, bacteria, and mushrooms. Beta-D-glucans stimulate the body's macrophages and other immune system weaponry to arrest cancer or tumor initiation, growth,

Stuffed Shiitake Mushrooms

Shiitake mushrooms (as well as also-medicinal maitake and—much less tasty—reishi mushrooms) have immune-boosting properties that help prevent the body from forming cancer cells. Though these mushrooms do not grow wild in the U.S., they are so widely cultivated that most people can easily find a locally grown source. While potent shiitake extracts are available in capsule form, research suggests that eating cooked shiitakes is a good way to reap the mushrooms' health benefits as well. Shiitakes with a rounded shape are much easier to stuff. Be sure to remove every last bit of the tough stems. **Serves 4 as an appetizer.**

Ingredients
- 3 tablespoons olive oil, divided
- ½ cup onion, minced
- 3 cloves garlic, minced
- ½ cup red bell pepper, minced
- ½ cup whole-grain breadcrumbs
- ½ cup Parmesan cheese, shredded
- 2 tablespoons fresh flat-leaf parsley, chopped
- ¼ teaspoon dried oregano
- ¼ teaspoon dried basil
- ½ teaspoon salt
- 16 medium shiitake mushrooms, stems removed

Directions: Preheat oven to 350 degrees. In a medium pan, heat 1 tablespoon olive oil over medium heat. Sauté onion, garlic, and bell pepper for five to 10 minutes, until onions are soft and beginning to brown.

Remove onion mixture from heat and add to a mixing bowl with breadcrumbs, cheese, parsley, spices, and salt. Add remaining olive oil as needed to moisten mixture. Stir to combine.

Place shiitakes on an oiled baking sheet and stuff each mushroom with the filling, pressing with a spoon.

Bake 20 minutes, until mushrooms are tender and filling is hot. Serve warm.

Amy Mayfield

Sautéed Shiitake and Bok Choy

Rev up your immune system with this simple dish. Maitake mushrooms can be used as a substitute.

Ingredients
- 1 teaspoon olive oil
- 1 large clove garlic, finely chopped
- 2½ cups Chinese bok choy, sliced into 1-inch segments
- ⅔ cup green onions, sliced
- 1⅓ cups fresh shiitake mushrooms, caps only, washed and sliced
- 2 tablespoons shoyu soy sauce
- Steamed rice, Belgian endive, and sliced avocado

Directions: Heat oil in a skillet and cook garlic on medium-high for about one minute.

Add bok choy, green onions, mushrooms, and soy sauce, and sauté for two to three minutes until the bok choy greens are wilted.

Serve with steamed rice, a few endive leaves, and sliced avocado.

Gina Mohammed

---

and spread. They also thwart bacterial, parasitic, and viral pathogens, including those of AIDS and hepatitis B.

Is eating the mushroom itself as effective as taking lentinan extract? In a therapeutic sense, probably not, since levels found in whole foods typically are lower and more variable than from controlled botanical extracts. But long-term benefits can accrue by eating the mushrooms as a component of a balanced diet, especially considering that shiitakes (and other medicinal mushrooms) contain minerals, vitamins, proteins, and other beneficial chemicals, including linoleic acid and ergosterol, which help lower cholesterol and the risk of arteriosclerosis.

Marvelous Maitake

Maitake (*Grifola frondosa*), also known as "dancing mushroom," might have gotten its name from a time long ago when people who found them reputedly danced for joy—not surprising, considering these treasures were worth their weight in silver. Found in the northern temperate forests of Asia and Europe, eastern Canada and the northeastern U.S.—and cultivated increasingly in North America—maitake is much in demand by chefs and gourmands for its sublime taste and texture, and its distinctive, earthy aroma.

It is equally pursued for its medicinal prowess.

Maitake, like shiitake, is an immune booster and cancer fighter. Extracts of its beta-D-glucans administered with whole maitake powder and standard chemotherapy promoted cancer regression or significant symptom improvement in 58 percent of liver cancer patients, 69 percent of breast cancer patients, and 62 percent of lung cancer patients (but much less in patients with leukemia, stomach cancer, or brain cancer), according to a 2002 report in *Alternative Medicine Review*. Other clinical studies show that the extracts increase production of interleukin-12, which activates the body's natural killer cells. Many additional benefits have been indicated for maitake, including possible regulation of cholesterol, diabetes, high blood pressure, viral infection, and liver disease.

The Role of Reishi

A rare find in the wild, the Asian reishi (*Ganoderma lucidum*) mushroom is so bitter you won't want to bite into its cap. And even if you tried, it would be too woody. In fact, reishi's polished hardness and bonsai-evoking appearance has made it a prized shelf ornament. But its medicinal properties have won many North American fans, who readily acquire imported reishi from China. The mushroom is traditionally sliced and simmered for tea or boiled in soups, then the pieces are discarded.

Reishi's bitter properties are due to its rich supply of terpenoids, elite

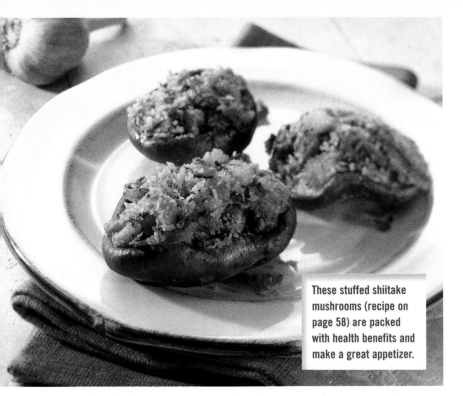

These stuffed shiitake mushrooms (recipe on page 58) are packed with health benefits and make a great appetizer.

plant chemicals that can work as antioxidants, immune-system stimulants, blood pressure regulators, and anticholesterol agents. Reishi's terpenoids include ganoderic acid, ganaderiol, and lucidumol, all with antiviral properties. Together with its other constituents—coumarins, which are natural blood thinners; phospholipids, which are anti-inflammatory and nerve protective; and the beta-D-glucans—reishi stocks a comprehensive medicinal cabinet that may well render it the mushroom of choice for health.

Dried reishi powder has been a popular anticancer agent in China since ancient times. A review in *Integrative Cancer Therapies* indicates that it deters even highly invasive breast and prostate cancer cells from spreading and becoming established in the body. And a clinical study from *Immunological Investigations* found that patients with advanced-stage cancer showed improvements in their immune responses when treated with reishi polysaccharide extracts for 12 weeks.

Even in healthy people, reishi boosts antioxidant capacity, as demonstrated in a recent study published in the *International Journal of Food Sciences and Nutrition*. This study showed that patients receiving either 10-day supplementation with encapsulated reishi (0.72 grams daily, equivalent to about 6.6 grams of fresh mushroom) or a single dose of 1.1 grams had an acute spike in plasma antioxidant capacity, without apparent toxic effects.

As an aid to healthy aging and longevity, reishi also helps detoxify the liver, prevent arteriosclerosis, and manage Alzheimer's disease (for which a Japanese reishi product has been patented). Other studies demonstrate anti-allergic, anti-inflammatory, and antibacterial actions—and the research continues. With all these dividends, reishi may be one bitter pill you will want to swallow.

Getting the Best

These special mushrooms are available fresh, dried, canned, powdered, or in extracted forms from supermarkets, health-food stores, and mail-order sources. As a general health supplement, try a daily serving of about 5 grams of dried reishi or maitake (about one medium mushroom) or 5 to 15 grams dried shiitake (one to three mushrooms).

For best results, remember these tips when buying and using medicinal mushrooms:

• Before using dried mushrooms, soak them in lightly salted or sugared hot water or stock for about an hour. Powders and extracts should be used according to package instructions and the advice of your health-care provider. (Mushrooms can interact with some over-the-counter and prescription drugs. Check with your health-care provider before taking.)

• Store fresh mushrooms in paper bags in the coldest part of your refrigerator, and eat them within seven days of purchase. Canned mushrooms last about a year, while dried ones sealed in plastic and stored in the freezer can last indefinitely.

• If possible, choose mushrooms grown on natural wood logs rather than sawdust. You will pay more for log-cultured mushrooms, but they tend to taste better, last longer, and shrink less during cooking. Their medicinal quality should be better, too.

Tough Living Makes Mighty Medicine

Why are medicinal mushrooms so gifted? Their strength comes from doing one of the most arduous jobs in nature—digesting dead or dying hardwood trees like oaks, elms, and plums. Shiitake, maitake, and reishi are wood composters that infiltrate tough tree trunks and roots using threadlike fingers, called mycelium, to digest and recycle nutrients back to the forest floor for the next generation of plants. Mushrooms are the fruit bodies that sprout when growing conditions are sufficiently cool and moist.

To do their job, these fungi must outcompete other fungi and microbes while dismantling the vast chemical complex of the tree. They must be aggressive yet defensive, a feat accomplished through biochemical combat. Harvested mushrooms possess potent bioactive chemicals, as well as nutrients gleaned from the tree. The button mushrooms commonly sold in supermarkets are far less competitive in nature and less active medicinally. 🌿

Gina Mohammed, Ph.D., is a plant physiologist living in Sault Ste. Marie, Ontario, Canada.

Chaga's Charm

One mighty mushroom can keep you healthy all winter long.

By Susanna Raeven

Chaga mushroom (*Inonotus obliquus*), the birch loving mushroom that does not look like one, is an ancient remedy that has been valued for its many health benefits for centuries. You will find it while walking through temperate forests looking for encrusted black formations on wounded or dying white birch trees. The sterile and cork-like mycelium grows out of remaining tree cavities after storms and other impacts break branches. A tree and its chaga companion can coexist for many years, and the mushroom can be harvested several times over the course of time.

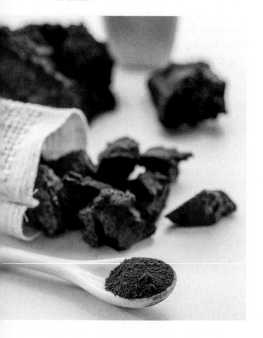

Health Benefits of Chaga

Most of the medical research on chaga has been done in Russia where the mushroom grows in abundance as it prefers cold climate forests. Chaga mushroom is an adaptogen. Adaptogenic plants and mushrooms help to bring the body back into balance and have beneficial effects on the nervous system, immune system, the GI tract, the cardiovascular system, and the endocrine system. Adaptogens help us to cope with stress, stay healthy during the cold and flu season, fight cancer, and lift us out of the dark depths of depression and adrenal burnout. They have immune-modulating properties that make them helpful in treating auto-immune diseases and have high levels of antioxidants that protect cells from damaging free radicals. Adaptogens gently tone and support the body systems over time and need to be taken for a minimum of two months to develop the full effect of their healing powers. Enjoying a cup of chaga tea daily during the fall and winter months ensures you are receiving support when it is needed most.

Chaga mushroom tea has a pleasant and slightly bitter taste with a hint of vanilla; it reminds me of a blend between strong black tea and coffee (without the nervous jitter as it does not contain caffeine or any other stimulants). I enjoy it very much with almond or hazelnut milk, and sweetened with a touch of maple syrup or honey.

It is an excellent alternative for people suffering from ulcers or adrenal fatigue who have to stop drinking coffee.

I always have a pot of chaga on the back of my stove during the winter months. It is my daily warming power beverage on winter days when my energy is turned inward and I spend most of my time inside. Tasting chaga evokes in me the sweet memory of the lush forest in summer time and reminds me to feel gratitude for the woods surrounding us, now sleeping under a thick blanket of snow. The crushed chaga chunks can be boiled over and over again until the raven black color of the tea finally starts to fade. Then a fresh chaga batch can be brewed by adding a few new chunks to the water. Chaga is sterile and antibacterial; I have never encountered chaga tea fermenting, even after sitting on the stove for many days. 🌿

Susanna Raeven is an herbalist, medicinal herb grower, and owner of Raven Crest Botanicals.

Chaga Chai

This chai is deliciously sweet, warming, and spicy. You can add other spices. Be creative and make small batches until you find the spice mix you like most. You can also add medicinal herb roots to your blend such as astragalus, burdock, or eleuthreo.

Ingredients
- 4 ounces chaga chunks or powder
- 1 teaspoon maca powder
- 2 teaspoons cinnamon back chips
- 2 teaspoons dried orange peel
- 1 teaspoon dried rose hips
- 1 teaspoon cardamom pods
- 1 teaspoon cardamom seeds or powder
- 1 tablespoon fresh ginger, thinly sliced

Directions: Blend dry herbs together and store in an airtight jar. Boil 4 tablespoons of the chaga blend together with the fresh ginger in 1 quart water until raven black.

Strain and serve with almond milk and optional honey or maple syrup. Boil same blend at least 10 times.

Oregon Grape

This beautiful ornamental is high in antioxidants and may treat psoriasis.

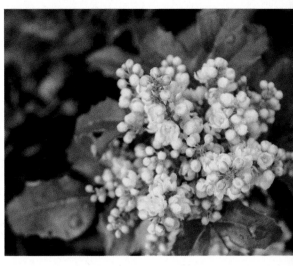

By Betsy Strauch

Good autumn leaf color, abundant clusters of yellow flowers, and blue-black, edible fruits have made Oregon grape a widely promoted ornamental, especially in the American West. Less well known are its coloring and medicinal properties, which have long been used by Native Americans and others.

A handsome spiny-leaved evergreen shrub, Oregon grape (*Mahonia aquifolium*) is native to western North America from British Columbia to Northern California but is planted throughout much of the country. It grows to about 6 feet tall and 3 to 5 feet wide and spreads by suckers.

The dense clusters of tiny flowers, which appear in March through May, are 2 to 3 inches long and slightly fragrant; they're Oregon's state flower. Grapelike berries ⅓ inch in diameter ripen in July through September and are the source of the plant's common names, Oregon grape holly and Oregon holly grape.

Hardy in Zones 4 or 5 to 8, it's best grown in the shade in hotter climates and with protection from leaf-scorching winter winds in colder ones. 'Compacta' is a 2-foot-tall cultivar with foliage that starts out glossy light green and turns to a dull green in summer. For a ground cover, try 10-inch-tall creeping mahonia (*M. repens*), which has dull blue-green leaves in summer and smaller "grapes."

Medicinal Uses

The fruits are high in vitamin C and have been used to treat and prevent scurvy, but the bitter roots and root bark are the parts usually used in medicinal preparations. Native American medicine men prescribed them to stimulate the appetite as well as to treat ulcers, heartburn, rheumatism, and kidney and skin disorders. White settlers learned about these uses and invented more of their own: a nineteenth-century remedy for hemorrhage and jaundice was made by steeping the roots in hot beer. The alternative common name yerba de sangre ("blood herb") testifies to its use as a blood purifier. It is mildly laxative.

Much of Oregon grape's current use seems based on tradition or on limited studies of its primary active ingredient, the alkaloid berberine, which is also found in other *Mahonia* species, barberry and goldenseal. Berberine stimulates the flow of bile, supporting its use to improve gall bladder function, and kills bacteria and amoebas, which seems to support its use in Asia to treat diarrhea. Oregon grape is high in antioxidants, compounds that neutralize the cell-damaging free radicals implicated in many diseases. A study showing that alkaloids found in Oregon grape slowed division of certain skin cells, together with its antioxidant activity, suggest its usefulness for treating psoriasis, a chronic inflammatory disease characterized by overproduction of skin cells.

Growing It

Oregon grape prefers well-drained, humus-rich soil and a spot in the shade, but it will tolerate less-than-ideal conditions. Established plants need little water except in the South. Shape plants by pruning long stalks out at the base and removing unwanted suckers.

The species may be propagated from seeds. Fresh seeds (with the flesh removed) germinate readily. Chilling for three months in moist planting medium enhances more rapid germination. Keep the seedlings in a nursery bed for a year, then transplant to their permanent locations.

To propagate cultivars, either divide entire plants, dig up some of the suckers, or root stem cuttings taken in summer or fall (dip the lower ends in rooting hormone). Any of these methods may also be used to increase your stock of the species.

The herb's typical pests include rusts, aphids, scales, and whiteflies. A looper caterpillar that sometimes disfigures the leaves can be tamed by applying the biological control Bacillus thuringiensis. Chlorosis (yellowing of the leaves) may occur in alkaline soils and probably indicates the need for a plant that's better adapted to those conditions.

Harvest the roots in late fall or early spring. 🌿

Betsy Strauch was a writer for *The Herb Companion*.

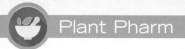

Grow, Cook, Heal with
Elderberries

This herbal shrub bears tasty blossoms and berries that can fight colds and flu.

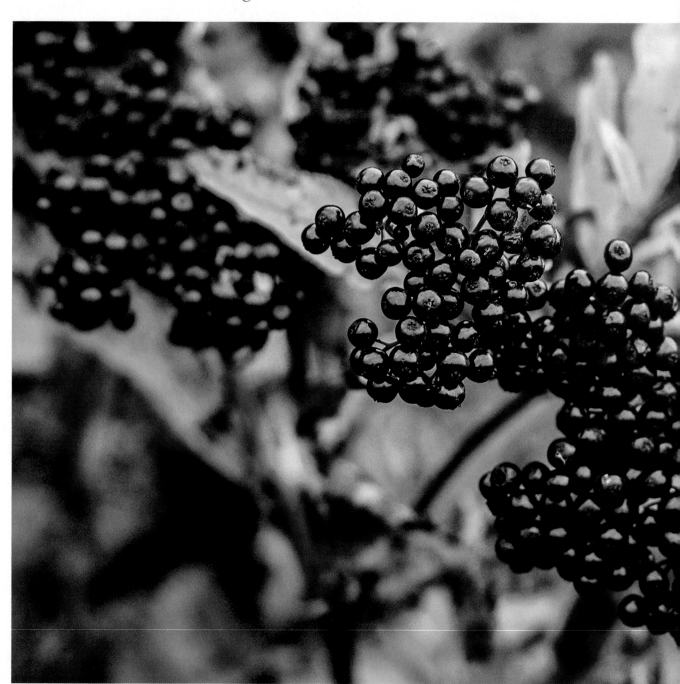

By Margie Gibson

Certain flavors, like scents, can simply transport you. Shortly after I moved to Bavaria, I settled in at a window table in a restaurant in southern Germany with a glass of golden Sekt sparkling wine. A splash of elderflower syrup had been added, and each sip sparked memories of my childhood: gathering elder blossoms with my grandmother on an early summer day in the hills of central Missouri; sitting next to my grandfather at the table, digging into a plate of warm elderflower pancakes; cutting clusters of elderberries in early autumn to make delicious syrup for winter.

Throughout the Werdenfelser region of Bavaria, elder bushes herald the arrival of summer with clusters of lacy white flowers. It's impossible to miss the plants. The umbels of tiny, five-petaled flowers produce a subtle but unmistakable scent. When the berries begin to form several weeks later, the blossoms drift softly to the ground like snowflakes. By early autumn, the shrubs are covered with heavy clusters of nutritious berries.

Elder is indigenous to broad stretches of the Northern Hemisphere —from North America, Europe, and Asia, and into North Africa along the Mediterranean coast. In North America, the native species is *Sambucus canadensis*, commonly called American elder; its European relative is *S. nigra*, know as European elder or black elder. Although both have served as a medicine chest for millennia, you'll find elder's flavor reason enough to hunt down a shrub for making delicious treats with its berries and blossoms. Don't want to walk a country mile for your elder? This shrub is easy to grow.

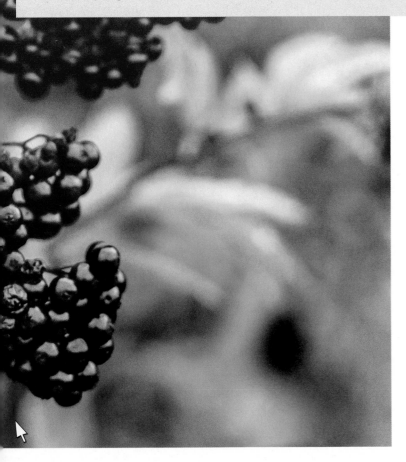

Elder Medicine

The plant has sustained generations as a source of food and medicine. Archaeologists found elder seeds in a Neolithic dwelling in Switzerland, and European villagers have planted the shrubs close to their homes for many centuries. Throughout North America, native tribes ate the dried berries as a winter staple, used the twigs and fruit in basketry, and used the branches to make arrows and musical instruments. Native Americans also used elderflowers and berries to treat colds, joint pain, fever, skin problems, and more.

All parts of the elder plant—flowers, bark, berries, and leaves—have been used medicinally. Modern research supports the use of elder syrup as a treatment for coughs and colds. According to the USDA, elderberries are exceptionally rich in vitamin C and antioxidants, which enhance the immune system. The flowers contain flavonoids and rutin, which also are known to improve immune function, especially in combination with vitamin C. In addition, lab studies have shown elderberries have significant anti-inflammatory and antiviral abilities. In clinical trials, patients taking elderberry extract recovered from the flu earlier, and had less severe symptoms, than patients in a control group.

The German word for elder, *holunder* (*holler*, in Southern German dialects), originates in pre-Christian legends. In the ancient Germanic pantheon, the goddess of life and death, Frau Holle, lived in the elder tree. Of course, any tree with such an illustrious resident would generate many traditions and stories. In one tale, men raised their hats when passing by an elder bush to honor Frau Holle. According to another story, a gardener or farmer had to request Frau Holle's permission to cut back an elder bush, or bad luck would result.

Easy-Growing Elder

Although elder grow wild throughout much of the U.S. and Canada, you won't have to hunt for the plant if you grow it yourself. Fall or early spring are ideal planting times. The shrub can survive as far north as Zone 3, and by its second year, will provide you with scented white blossoms in late May to late June, followed by huge clusters of berries in late August to early October, depending on your location.

Elder is easy to grow in either full sun or

Elderflower Syrup

Ingredients
- Elderflowers (enough to loosely fill a ½-gallon jar), rinsed and cleaned
- 2 lemons, washed and sliced
- 4⅛ cups water
- 5½ cups sugar
- 1 packet (50 grams) citric acid

Directions: Stuff flowers and lemon slices into a large glass container with a lid. You should have enough flowers to almost fill the jar.

To make syrup, bring water to a boil in a 2-quart saucepan, then add sugar and boil several minutes. Remove pan from heat, let cool; stir in citric acid.

Pour syrup over flowers and lemon slices. Close jar and let sit in a sunny spot for 2 or 3 days.

Remove flowers and lemon slices, but first squeeze out their flavored syrup. Bottle syrup in clean glass jars with tight lids. Store in refrigerator. **Makes about 3 pints.**

Elderflower Liqueur

Ingredients for liqueur
- 12 ounces elderflowers, rinsed and cleaned
- 3 ounces fresh lemon balm leaves, rinsed
- Peel of 3 lemons (avoid the bitter white pith)
- ½ liter vodka
- 2 cups sugar syrup (use less if you want the final drink to be less sweet)

Ingredients for sugar syrup
- 2 cups water
- 1 cup sugar

Directions: Stuff elder blossoms, lemon balm, and lemon peel into a clean glass jar. Pour vodka over herbs and press down so vodka covers everything. Let jar sit on countertop for 1 month. Shake once a day; vodka gradually will turn deep amber in color.

After a month, remove herbs and lemon peel. Squeeze them over a large bowl to remove flavored vodka. Strain vodka in the jar through a sieve into the same bowl. Thoroughly clean the jar, then return flavored vodka to the jar.

To make sugar syrup, bring water to a boil. Add sugar, return to boil, and simmer until liquid is clear. Remove from heat and cool.

Add cooled sugar syrup to jar, cover, and let sit for another 2 weeks. After 2 weeks, pour liqueur into small, decorative bottles and seal.

To serve, pour a portion into a small container and chill in the freezer until very cold. Serve in chilled cordial glasses. **Makes 4 cups.**

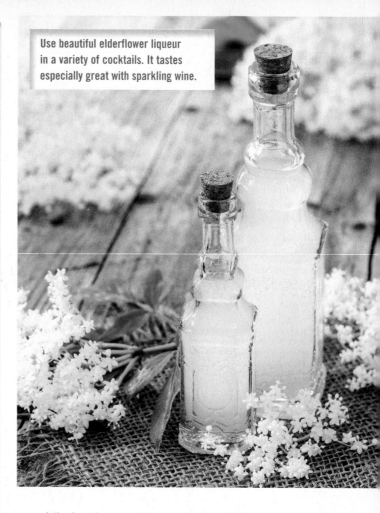

Use beautiful elderflower liqueur in a variety of cocktails. It tastes especially great with sparkling wine.

partial shade. Choose at least two bushes of the same variety to ensure bigger yields of blooms and berries, and plant 6 to 10 feet apart in well-drained, fertile soil with a pH between 5.5 and 6.5. Work compost into the soil before planting to add nutrients and help retain moisture—in nature, elder thrives in moist woodland soil and along stream banks. The shrub's root system is shallow, so tamp the soil firmly in place after planting, and avoid using a cultivator around the shrub; instead, pull weeds by hand. Elder thrives on about an inch of water weekly. If your area doesn't receive that much rainfall, you'll need to help out.

You won't need to prune at all the first two years. In late winter or early spring of the third year, remove any broken or dead canes. To encourage new growth in subsequent years, cut back the oldest canes, which produce less fruit. Any cane more than three years old should be pruned, but try to keep equal numbers of 1-, 2- and 3-year-old canes.

Elder bushes are rarely troubled by plant diseases and pests, but birds love the ripe berries. To increase your own harvest, cover your elder with bird netting just as the berries begin to turn color.

Using Elder in Culinary Pursuits

Because elder grows so abundantly near my present home in Germany, I still collect the blossoms and berries from the wild (after asking Frau Holle's permission, of course). Last June, I headed out in search of the blossoms, toting a cotton bag perfect for foraging expeditions. I came across two huge, fragrant bushes where the gathering was easy. I quickly collected enough blossoms to make syrup, and plucked a few petals from some nearby wild roses to add to the elderflowers. As soon as I got home, I stuffed

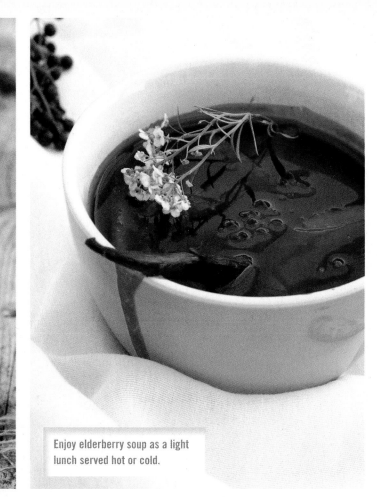
Enjoy elderberry soup as a light lunch served hot or cold.

Elderberry Soup with Semolina Dumplings

This soup could be served as a light lunch or dessert, and can be presented hot or cold, although I prefer it hot. If plums aren't in season, try another tart fruit such as gooseberries or cranberries.

When using elderberries for food or health, use only ripe black fruit; the red berries of a related species are poisonous.

Ingredients for soup

- 4¼ cups elderberry juice
- Squirt of lemon juice, plus a few pieces of lemon zest
- ½ cup sugar
- 4 cloves
- 1 stick cinnamon
- 10 Damson plums, halved and pitted
- 4 pears, peeled and sliced

Ingredients for dumplings

- 1 cup milk
- 1 tablespoon butter
- 2 teaspoons sugar
- ½ teaspoon vanilla extract
- Pinch of salt
- ⅔ cup semolina or Cream of Wheat
- 1 egg

Directions: In a large soup pot or Dutch oven, bring juices, sugar, cloves, and cinnamon to a boil, then reduce heat and simmer 10 minutes at a low temperature.

Add plums and pears; continue cooking until soft. Meanwhile, in a separate saucepan, combine milk, butter, sugar, vanilla, and salt; bring to a simmer.

While stirring constantly and cooking over low heat, sprinkle in semolina and cook until mixture thickens. Beat egg in a bowl, then add some of the semolina mixture to the egg.

Gradually add egg mixture back into pan with the rest of the semolina, stirring vigorously so egg doesn't curdle from heat. Remove pan from heat.

Using a teaspoon, make small dumplings from the semolina mixture. Bring a pot of salted water to boil, then gently drop in the dumplings. Cook about 5 minutes, or until dumplings rise to the top.

To serve, divide dumplings into bowls and add hot soup. **Serves 4 to 6.**

the blossoms and petals into a glass container, poured in sugar-water syrup, then put the container on the kitchen windowsill. After several days, I strained out the spent blossoms and bottled the rest — enough for a year's worth of Sekt.

A few days later, I was back on the hunt. This time, with a different recipe in mind: I wanted to create holundercello — a local version of limoncello, the sweet digestif of Italy's Amalfi coast. I collected another bag of blossoms, then put them in the glass jar along with a bundle of lemon balm and the peels of some organic lemons from a local market, then covered it all with vodka. After a month, the vodka turned deep amber and took on a wonderful blend of flavors and scents. I removed the herbs and added sugar syrup to the flavored vodka. After steeping for two more weeks, the holundercello was ready to serve chilled in small crystal glasses.

In late summer, I returned once more. This time to gather clusters of purple-black berries for jam, sauce, and soup. Now during the cold days of winter, I sip my own elder blossom Sekt and elderberry soup, warmed by the memories of gathering the flowers and fruit on sunny summer and early autumn days. 🌿

Margie Gibson writes about food, culture, history, and natural history. Previously, she worked at the Smithsonian National Zoological Park, where she wrote about wildlife.

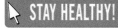

DO-IT-YOURSELF COUGH DROPS

Find relief from that wracking cough with these three herbal throat soothers.

By K.C. Compton and Susan Melgren

Coughing spells can attack us when we least expect it. So if you don't like the taste of store-bought cough drops, the bright color they leave your tongue, and the extra additives found in most—or if you're looking for a way to save money—make your own. With a few common household items and standout herbs, it's easy to get started.

Natural Throat Relievers

Horehound *(Marrubium vulgare)*, a natural cough suppressant and expectorant, is one of the major ingredients in over-the-counter herbal cough drops such as Ricola. Although it has an old-fashioned-sounding name, and indeed, is probably the cough remedy with which our great-grandparents were most familiar, horehound has up-to-date value in fighting coughs, colds, and catarrh (mucus buildup). Horehound is in the mint family, so consider growing it in a container to keep the plant from taking over. It grows from seeds or starts. Sow seeds up to three weeks before the last frost and space plants about 10 inches apart. As with other mints, go easy on the water. Harvest the flowers and leaves for medicinal use.

According to the American Botanical Council, horehound has been in use as an expectorant cough remedy since ancient Egyptian times and has been an important herb in treating wheezing, chronic bronchitis, and whooping cough. The German Commission E, a regulatory body that governs herbal remedies in Germany, also approves horehound for loss of appetite and for intestinal concerns such as bloating and flatulence. Native people throughout North America have used it for centuries as a cold remedy, attesting to its universal effectiveness. An aromatic perennial, horehound is hardy and can be grown and harvested readily.

To make your own cough medicine, try our Do-It-Yourself Cough Drops (page 67), which are made with horehound. This recipe also uses honey, which has been used medicinally since ancient times. (Hippocrates recommended it for optimal health circa 400 B.C.) Honey is a demulcent that soothes irritated

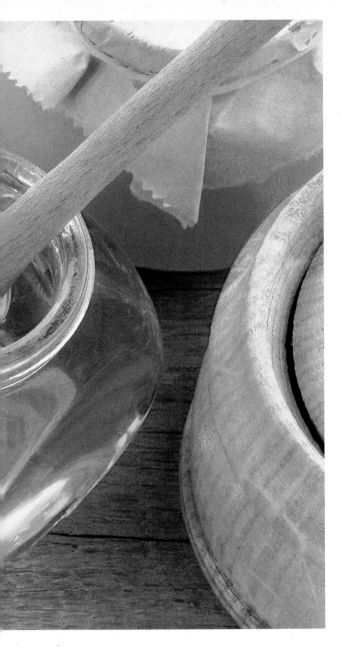

Do-It-Yourself Cough Drops

Here is a simple recipe that will fill a sandwich bag with golden horehound drops. Honey covers the bitter taste of this aromatic herb. You can substitute or combine with other herbs such as mint or sage.

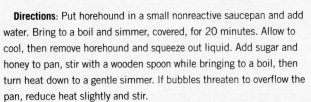

Ingredients

- 1 cup fresh horehound leaves
- 1 cup water
- 2 cups sugar
- 2 tablespoons honey
- Granulated or powdered sugar, to coat

Directions: Put horehound in a small nonreactive saucepan and add water. Bring to a boil and simmer, covered, for 20 minutes. Allow to cool, then remove horehound and squeeze out liquid. Add sugar and honey to pan, stir with a wooden spoon while bringing to a boil, then turn heat down to a gentle simmer. If bubbles threaten to overflow the pan, reduce heat slightly and stir.

Boil to hard-crack stage (330 degrees), but even if you use a candy thermometer, test often toward the end of cooking to get the hardness right. Keep a shallow cup of cold water nearby. Stir the liquid occasionally, and watch how it falls from the spoon. When it forms a thread, begin testing for hardness by allowing a drop of the mixture to fall into the cup of cold water. Don't trust your fingers to examine the now-hardened drop in the cup: Bite it. If it's at all gooey or sticks to your teeth, keep cooking. When it's hard enough to crack when you bite it, remove pan from heat immediately.

If the mixture crystallizes, just add a cup of water and an extra tablespoon of honey to the pan, scrape the crystalline chunks into it, and begin again.

Lightly butter a candy mold, cookie sheet, or other heatproof baking pan, and pour in the hot mixture. If you're using a flat-bottomed pan, score the surface of the candy after it has cooled enough to become firm. This will help in breaking it apart, which should be done as soon as the candy can be handled.

After individual drops are formed, sift granulated or powdered sugar over them to keep them from sticking together. Store in a moisture-proof container.

K.C. Compton

Sage Honey Syrup

This sage- and honey-infused syrup is delicious and makes a great herbal remedy for sore throats and tickly coughs.

Ingredients

- ¾ cup wildflower honey
- ¼ cup water
- 1 teaspoon lemon juice
- 1 tablespoon fresh sage, chopped

Directions: Stir all ingredients over medium heat until simmering. Remove from heat and let steep, covered, for 10 minutes.

Strain honey mixture and store in a sealed glass jar. Keeps in the refrigerator for up to three months.

Sarah Goldschmidt

mucus membranes and has been shown to reduce coughs better than dextromethorphan (the common over-the-counter cough suppressant) or a placebo. Do not give honey to children younger than 2.

Sage (*Salvia* spp.) is another herb that may help defend against aggravating coughs. Both the German Commission E and the USDA have deemed sage antibacterial, and the USDA even mentions white sage (*S. apiana*) as an acceptable treatment for sore throats because of its abilities to inhibit bacteria growth. Drink 1 cup of sage tea (steep 1 teaspoon of dried sage leaves, or 1 tablespoon fresh, in boiling water for three to five minutes) daily, or add 1 to 2 drops of essential oil to a glass of water. For a recipe, see Sage Honey Syrup at right. 🌿

K.C. Compton was a senior editor at *Mother Earth News*, and Susan Melgren was the web editor at *Mother Earth Living*.

Honey
& the History of Eating Your Medicine

Healing honey is a true miracle of nature. Learn more about honey's medicinal history, how you can use it to improve your family's health, and how to ensure you're buying from sustainable beekeepers.

By Dawn Combs

I'm still surprised when someone comes up to our farmers market booth and asks if there is any truth in the idea that honey is a health food. For me, a beekeeper and honey enthusiast for 10 years, it's difficult to imagine that people in the U.S. still think of honey as just a sweetener. Honey's many medicinal benefits have been employed throughout recorded history, and today we know more than ever about its scientifically backed healing properties.

History of Honey

In North America, the honeybee we know today was an import, brought with European settlers in the 17th century. Before that, this continent had native bees that did not collect as much honey. American Indians probably collected honey from wild hives, though we don't have much in the way of historical evidence.

The settlers who brought the bee here clearly understood her value. Yet at some point American culture came to doubt the medicinal quality of honey. Most likely this occurred when Western medicine came to the forefront and cast aspersions on folk healing. We are only now beginning to accept the value of honey as a medicine again with the help of modern medical studies that are returning honey to the hospital for the treatment of diabetic sores and burns, and into medicated bandages for everyday cuts.

Despite our forgetfulness here in the West, the worldwide use of honey as medicine has continued uninterrupted since ancient times. In Egypt, honey figured prominently in the maintenance of life and preparations for death. In ancient Greece, Hippocrates used it as a base for most of his formulations, a practice continued in the works of the medical greats such as Galen and Dioscorides. We have more than 4,000 years of recorded use of honey as medicine from the ancient world to the present. It has even been successfully used as battlefield medicine from the time of *The Iliad* to as recently as World War I.

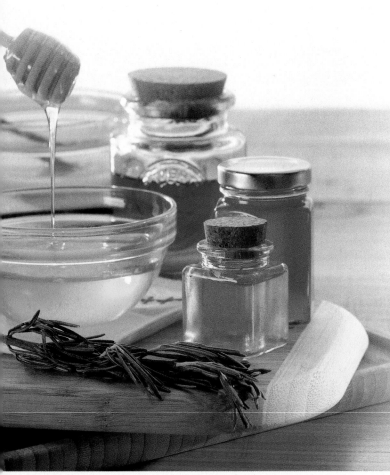

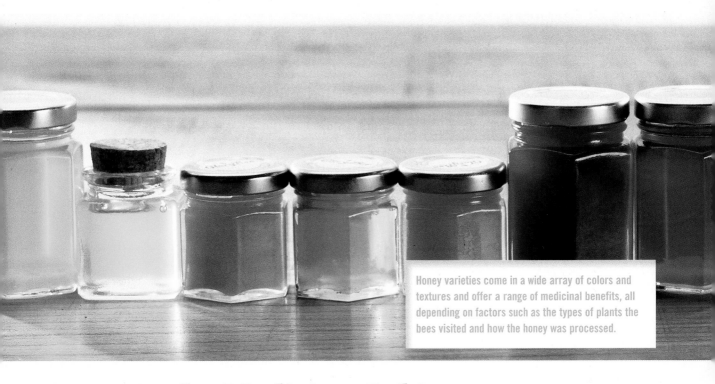

Honey varieties come in a wide array of colors and textures and offer a range of medicinal benefits, all depending on factors such as the types of plants the bees visited and how the honey was processed.

Honey in the Medicine Cabinet

Try these effective ways to use honey to heal everyday ailments.

ALLERGIES: Just a teaspoon a day of raw, local honey can decrease symptoms or prevent them altogether. For best results, start this regimen a month before your symptoms typically start to appear.

ARTHRITIS: It may be the alkalinizing effect of a mixture of honey and vinegar that seems to relieve the pain and inflammation of arthritis when used over a period of time. This mix is anti-inflammatory, used internally or externally.

CONJUNCTIVITIS (PINK EYE): Combine equal parts warm water and honey; stir to mix well. Allow the mix to cool, then apply as an eye wash. Be aware that honey can sting a bit.

COUGH: Mix equal parts vinegar and honey, and add a twist of lemon. Drink a bit of this mixture every two to three hours.

CUTS: A dab of honey underneath a bandage may serve you better than any antibiotic cream on the market.

DIABETIC SORES: Honey is one of the only treatments that can help an unresponsive diabetic wound. Apply directly to the sore and cover with light gauze.

DIAPER RASH: No matter how bad the rash, honey was always the best remedy for my kids. Just a thin coating and a bit of naked time and it healed up like magic.

DIARRHEA: Because it has a balancing effect on digestion, honey is useful for relieving both diarrhea and constipation.

IMMUNE SUPPORT: Routine eating of raw honey increases B-lymphocytes and T-lymphocytes, two types of white blood cells that improve immunity.

INSOMNIA: A spoonful of honey before bed can help support a good night's rest.

LEG CRAMPS: A mix of honey and vinegar rubbed onto the legs before bed increases circulation and can help prevent leg cramps.

MINOR BURNS: Spread honey liberally over the damaged skin of a burn and leave it open to the air. It's best not to apply anything more than a very light gauze.

NASAL CONGESTION: Add honey to a steam or simply spread it over the sinus areas on the face. Sinus congestion will drain quickly—be ready!

SINUSITIS: Add a teaspoon to a cup of saline water and use it in a neti pot. Never use a neti pot while you are congested.

SORE THROAT: Let a spoonful of honey melt in your mouth or drink it in a cup of hot tea for fast relief from an itching and scratching throat.

STOMACH ULCER: Honey inhibits *Helicobacter pylori*, the culprit behind most ulcers; eat 2 to 3 ounces a day for three months.

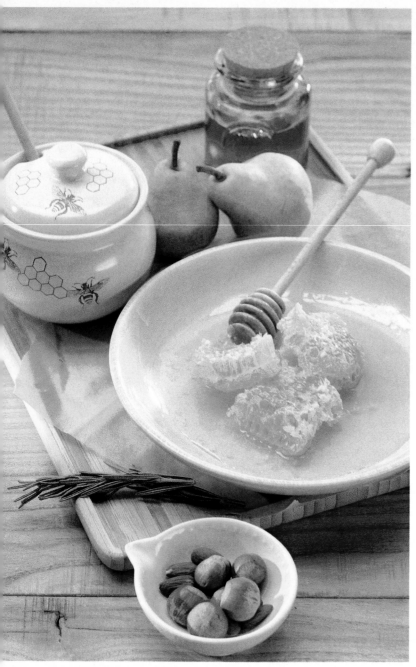
Honey contains the benefits of the original plant from which the nectar was collected.

on "supercharged" levels of certain nutrients and beneficial phytochemicals.

In the past several years, manuka honey has become popular. While this honey is every bit as fabulous as the marketing would have us believe, it's not unique in its medicinal fortitude. We demonstrate our lack of understanding of the honeybee when we fail to see the complexity of the honeys she creates. To the bee, nectar isn't mere sugar. Each flower has a varied vitamin and mineral content, so she is really filling her larder with a balanced diet just as we do with our grains, beans, vegetables, and dairy. Our shopping lists may also include items to soothe a headache, protect against infection, or relieve a cold. Each plant a bee visits has a different phytochemical profile, which allows her to mix her own medicine as well.

In the case of manuka honey, scientists have analyzed the honey that is collected from a specific tree (the manuka tree or *Leptospermum scoparium*) and found that it has an especially high mineral content and antibacterial activity. Interestingly, the manuka is in the same family as the Melaleuca group, which gives us the well-known antibacterial, tea tree oil.

Although manuka is indisputably medicinal, it is important to understand that every culture around the world has had its highly medicinal honeys. In Greece, there is an abundance of thyme honey, while sage, rosemary, or lavender honey may be found in other regions of the world. They all contain the benefits of the original plant from which the nectar was collected and can contain phytochemicals that are nourishing and relaxing to the nervous system, protect against fungal overgrowth, and much more.

Here in the U.S., one of our most medicinal honeys, buckwheat honey, is very dark and contains high levels of minerals and antibacterial activity, just like manuka honey. It has a rich, molasses-like taste that can be difficult for some people to get used to. Knowing that all well-raised, chemical-free, raw honey has medicinal benefits can free you up to be choosy and splurge on an imported honey, or simply convince you to buy from your local beekeeper instead.

Types of Honey

Perhaps some of the reason people doubt the truth of honey's healing powers lies in its variability. We still believe honey is honey. We know that it is antibacterial, but when someone in one part of the world touts honey as a cure-all for chest congestion, we doubt this lofty assertion rather than observing that their honey is collected in a grove of eucalyptus trees.

Lab tests show that various types of honey differ in their amounts of vitamins and minerals because every honey sample is made up of a different compilation of nectars. Depending which plants bees are visiting, honey can take

Bees' Needs

Understanding the complex nature of honey helps us better understand the bee and her needs. Scientists are studying the current disappearance of our bees, yet they often fail to consider bees' basic needs before entering the lab.

Bees that are trucked from one major monocrop field to another—the common practice in commercial farming—are weakened. Almonds are quite healthy, but if you ate only almonds day in and day out, you would be very sick.

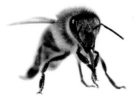

Only recently are we seeing growers in these large monoculture systems begin to allow native weeds and medicinal plants to grow in windrows to provide alternative forage for pollinators. As an interesting note, in an article recently published in *The New York Times*, biologist Mark Winston says, thanks to increases in crop yields, farmers who plant their entire field would earn $27,000 in profit from the farm; those who left a third unplanted for bees to nest and forage would earn $65,000 on a farm of similar size.

We know bodies not fed a balanced diet need more medical care. When the bee is denied the means to remain healthy, she is prey to disease, pests, and fungus, and is too tired and sick to avoid crops that are sprayed or unacceptably modified. Taking care of the health of the bee is job one—and a vital one for all of us, considering bees pollinate at least 30 percent of the world's crops and 90 percent of our wild plants. We can't possibly obtain optimal health benefits from products made by unhealthy bees. Indeed, we may find it much more difficult to survive without healthy bees in our world. 🐝

Dawn Combs is the owner of Mockingbird Meadows Herbal Health Farm in central Ohio and the director of its Eclectic Herbal Institute (MockingbirdMeadows. com). Mockingbird Meadows is nationally known for its line of herbal honey spreads. Dawn is the author of *Sweet Remedies* and *Heal Local;* both books are available at MotherEarthNews.com/Store.

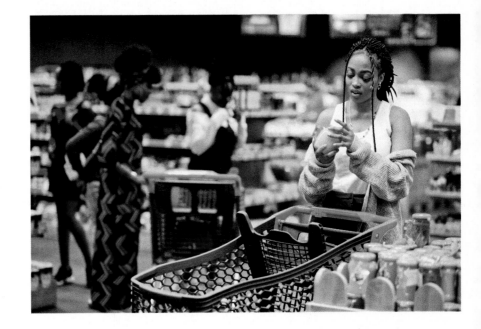

How to Buy Quality Honey

There is a myth that raw honey is solid. In truth, honey comes out of the comb as a liquid. Depending on the types of nectar and pollen, raw honey crystallizes at different speeds. There's no good way to know if honey is raw except to check the labels and ask your beekeeper. Here are some questions to guide your next healthful honey hunt.

1 **DO YOU USE CHEMICALS IN YOUR HIVES?** Make sure herbal or nonchemical methods are used.

2 **DO YOU HARVEST WITH AN ELECTRIC KNIFE?** Heated knives can superheat honey, decreasing healthy enzymes.

3 **HAS THE HONEY BEEN FILTERED?** Make sure only the largest particles are strained prior to bottling instead of applying pressure and heat.

4 **IS THE HONEY PASTEURIZED?** While pasteurizing makes honey clear for the store shelf, health and taste are lost.

5 **WHEN WAS YOUR HONEY HARVESTED?** For those allergic to spring pollens, spring varietals can provide better allergy protection. Or grab one harvested at the end of the previous season for a full array of pollen protection.

6 **HOW DO YOU RE-LIQUIFY YOUR HONEY?** Bucket heaters can overheat, so consider the speed at which honey is warmed for bottling.

7 **HOW DO YOU FEED YOUR BEES?** Many beekeepers feed bees high-fructose corn syrup or boiled sugar water. Find sustainable beekeepers who feed bees their own honey.

8 **WHERE ARE YOU?** Raw, local honey is best for allergies, but all raw honey is beneficial. There's no mileage limit for sellers to claim a "local" product, so make sure bees are collecting from the same plants as where you live.

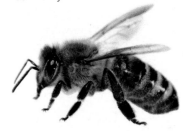

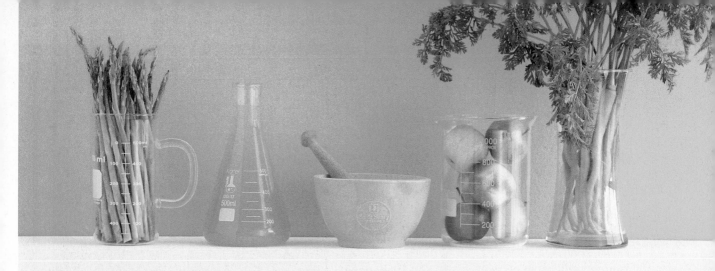

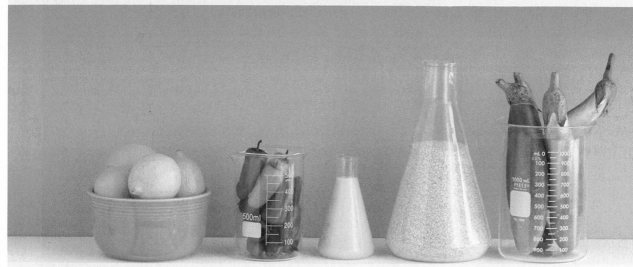

FIGHT ILLNESS WITH
THESE FOODS

Six pioneering doctors share their favorite recipes to naturally

boost your family's immunity — no drugstore needed.

By Tabitha Alterman

Enterovirus, ebola, swine flu — it seems as if every year there is a new crop of illnesses to worry about. Although it can be easy to fret when cold and flu season comes around, our best defense is in keeping our bodies strong with the power of a healthy diet. We have known about the healing powers of food since at least the time of the ancient Greek physician Hippocrates, who famously said, "Let food be thy medicine and medicine be thy food."

It's interesting that the father of Western medicine promoted an idea that it seems many Western medical practitioners —

often quicker to prescribe drugs than lifestyle habits — now seem to have lost a connection with. (Hippocrates also said, "Walking is man's best medicine.")

The medical professionals included in this article all stand with Hippocrates' wise counsel, and so they offer you a proactive prescription for winter illnesses in the form of delicious recipes and useful kitchen tips. Happy cooking, and here's to your health!

Tabitha Alterman is the author of *Feel-Good Superfoods*.

Medicinal Mushrooms

Many wild mushrooms have healing properties to support healthy immune function. Maitake and shiitake are two of the most powerful and abundant, as well as flavorful. The parsley, garlic, onion, and olive oil all add antioxidants to boost the power of this delicious side dish.

Ingredients
- 2 tablespoons extra virgin olive oil
- 2 cloves garlic, finely chopped
- 1 yellow onion, coarsely chopped
- 1 pound each of maitake and shiitake mushrooms, well rinsed and coarsely chopped
- ½ cup fresh Italian parsley, finely chopped (reserve some for garnish)
- ½ teaspoon sea salt

Directions: In a sauté pan, warm olive oil. Add garlic and onion, stirring occasionally until onion is slightly translucent.

Add mushrooms and sauté until slightly tender, about 10 minutes.

Remove from heat, mix in parsley, and season with salt to taste.

Transfer to serving bowl, garnish with remaining parsley, and enjoy!

Lawrence Rosen is the founder of The Whole Child Center, an integrative and ecologically sustainable pediatric practice in New Jersey, and co-author of Treatment Alternatives for Children. *Learn more at LawrenceRoseNMD.com.*

Spicy Mussels With Kale

With its combination of high mineral density, a burst of antioxidants from the chilies and kale, and a hefty dose of vitamin B12 and omega-3s, this dish is a winter essential for immune health. Our bodies' innate defense systems revolve around minerals such as selenium, manganese, and zinc—all abundant in this dish.

Ingredients
- 2 pounds tightly closed raw mussels
- 1 tablespoon olive oil
- 4 cloves garlic, thinly sliced
- 1 small chili, such as habanero or serrano, seeds removed, minced

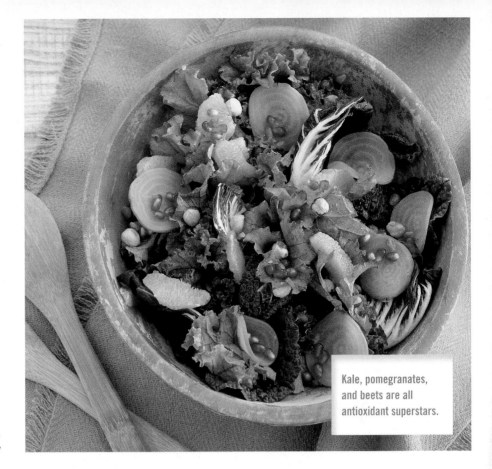

Kale, pomegranates, and beets are all antioxidant superstars.

- 1 bunch kale (about 10 ounces), trimmed and thinly sliced (makes about 10 cups)
- ½ cup white wine
- 1 pound diced tomatoes (about 3 medium tomatoes), or one 15-ounce can
- ¼ teaspoon salt
- ⅛ teaspoon freshly ground black pepper
- ¼ cup chopped fresh flat-leaf parsley

Directions: Soak mussels in a bowl of cold water for 15 to 20 minutes. Put mussels in a colander and rinse under cold running water several times. Discard any that are open. Check each mussel for a threadlike string hanging out of the shell (called the beard). To remove the beard, using a tea towel, take hold of the beard, pull firmly toward the hinge end of the shell, and tug it free.

Heat a large saucepan over medium-high heat. Add olive oil, garlic, and chili. Reduce heat to medium-low and cook for 1 minute, stirring occasionally until garlic becomes fragrant.

Add mussels, kale, wine, tomatoes, salt, and pepper. Cover and cook for 3 to 4 minutes more, shaking pan until mussels open and meat inside is cooked through. Discard any mussels that have not opened. Sprinkle with parsley and serve immediately.

Drew Ramsey is a Columbia University-trained psychiatrist who specializes in holistic brain health, nutrition, and integrative care. He is an assistant clinical professor of psychiatry at Columbia, a farmer, and author of The Happiness Diet *and* 50 Shades of Kale. *Learn more at DrewRamseyMD.com.*

Pomegranate Kale Winter Salad

With kale, pomegranates and beets, this superfood-filled salad is an antioxidant superstar. Make the dressing ahead of time, then whip up the salad just before serving.

Ingredients for Vinaigrette
- 1 small shallot, chopped
- Juice of 1 small tangerine
- 3 tablespoons ume plum vinegar
- ¼ cup balsamic vinegar
- 3 tablespoons pomegranate molasses (found at Mediterranean grocers)
- 2 tablespoons honey
- 2 tablespoons fresh herbs or fennel fronds
- A couple generous grinds of fresh cracked black pepper
- ½ cup extra virgin olive oil

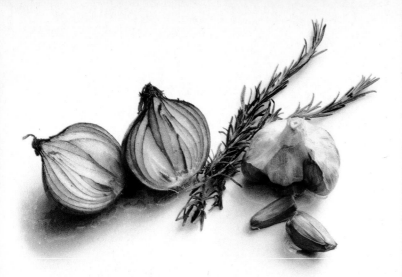

5 Food-Based Tips for a Strong Immune System

1. Eat garlic, onions, ginger, & lots of spices (such as oregano, turmeric, cinnamon, and sage).
Add spices and herbs to soups, stews, casseroles, meats, and vegetables, as well as bean dips and sauces. Garlic and onions offer wide-spectrum antimicrobial properties.

2. Eat many servings of colorful fruits and vegetables high in vitamins A, C, and phytonutrients that support the immune system.
Choose more leafy greens, cruciferous vegetables (broccoli, Brussels sprouts, cauliflower), peppers, sweet potatoes, and squashes. Aim for three to four servings of fruits and four or more servings of vegetables daily.

3. Drink plenty of fluids, especially warm fluids.
With drier air inside and out, winter can be a particularly challenging time to stay hydrated. Consuming adequate fluids supports all of our bodies' functions, including the immune system. Make soups and broths (from scratch with fresh vegetables is always best) and have them throughout the week. Drink teas made from warming herbs such as ginger and echinacea daily. Keep filtered water with you at all times. Avoid concentrated fruit juices and sweetened beverages, as the sugar content is harmful for the immune system.

4. Avoid simple sugars as much as possible.
This includes sweet treats and desserts but also the white flour and refined grain products that turn into sugar quickly. Studies have shown that refined sugars can suppress our immune systems for hours after ingested.

5. Have protein with each meal.
Proteins are the building blocks of the body. This includes our immune and detoxification systems. Organic, clean, and lean animal protein as well as plant-based (legumes, nuts/seeds) proteins are important to include in each meal and snack.

Ingredients for Salad
- 2 medium golden beets, sliced thin
- 1 pomegranate
- ¾ cup hazelnuts
- 1 bunch lacinato kale, washed, dried, torn into bite-size pieces
- 1 bunch green kale, washed, dried, torn into bite-size pieces
- Salt and pepper, to taste
- 1 medium fennel bulb, cut into thin strips
- 1 small head radicchio, sliced into ribbons
- 2 grapefruits, peeled, segmented

Directions for vinaigrette: Combine all ingredients except olive oil in blender or bowl for immersion blender.

With blender running, slowly add olive oil until vinaigrette has emulsified. Makes about 1¼ cups.

Directions for salad: Preheat oven to 350 F.

In a small pot of boiling water, blanch beet slices for 2 minutes. Set aside and let cool.

Slice pomegranate in half. Hold one half cut-side-down over a bowl. Use a wooden spoon to smack the back of the pomegranate, knocking arils into bowl.

Place hazelnuts on a cookie sheet and bake for about 15 minutes, shaking every 5 minutes until fragrant and skins loosen. Wrap in clean dish towel and rub skins off. Set aside.

To assemble salad, massage ¼ cup dressing into kale and sprinkle with salt and pepper.

Toss fennel with 2 tablespoons of dressing and scatter over kale.

Arrange remaining ingredients and add additional dressing as desired.

Chef Kendra Marable

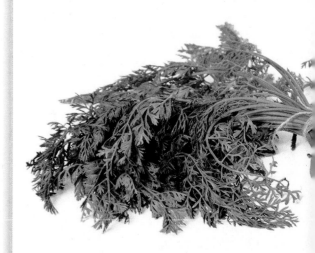

Ginger Carrot Soup

Ginger is a wonderful digestive aid that strengthens the lining of the gastrointestinal tract, protecting us against parasites. The carotenes in carrots fortify the immune system and help maintain healthy skin and hair. Carrots and ginger both pack a nutritional punch and, combined, they offer an incredible flavor.

When buying carrots, immediately remove the greens. They leach vitamins and moisture from the edible roots.

Ingredients
- 2 teaspoons grapeseed oil
- 1 medium onion, chopped
- 3 tablespoons fresh ginger root, peeled, finely chopped
- 3 cups chopped carrots
- 1 medium potato, peeled, chopped
- 8 cups vegetable stock
- Salt, to taste
- Dash of dry sherry
- Dash of ground nutmeg
- Fresh parsley or cilantro, chopped (optional)

Directions: Heat oil in a large pot. Add onion and ginger. Sauté, stirring, just until onion is translucent.

Add carrots, potato, and stock. Bring to a boil. Cover and reduce heat to boil gently until vegetables are tender, 30 to 45 minutes.

Purée soup with an immersion blender or in batches in a blender or food processor.

Add salt to taste, and flavor with sherry and nutmeg. Serve plain or garnished with parsley or cilantro.

Andrew Weil is a world-renowned leader and pioneer in the field of integrative medicine, a healing-oriented approach to health care that encompasses body, mind, and spirit. Adapted from DRWeil.com.

Winter's Natural Medicine Cabinet

Herbal Cough Syrup

Elderberry is a respiratory immune tonic. Anise is a respiratory antispasmodic. Echinacea prevents recurrence of coughs, and catnip is relaxing.

Ingredients
- Elderberry syrup
- Anise seed tincture
- Echinacea glycerite
- Catnip tincture

Directions: Mix equal parts of all ingredients, which are available at health-food stores.

To use, give ½ teaspoon to kids and 1 teaspoon to adults 4 to 6 times a day. Continue for up to a week. If there's a tendency for recurrent coughs, stay on it for several weeks.

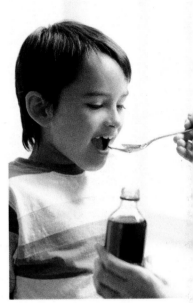

Aviva Romm is a Yale-trained physician specializing in integrative medicine for women and children, a midwife, herbalist, and author. Follow her at AvivaRomm.com or Facebook.com/AvivaRommMD.

Winter Elixir

Use this elixir daily throughout winter to keep your immune system functioning optimally. Astragalus is a deep immune tonic; eleuthero is an adaptogen; elderberry is a respiratory tonic with antiviral properties.

Ingredients
- 10 grams ashwagandha root
- 10 grams rhodiola root
- 10 grams astragalus root
- 150 milliliters brandy or vodka plus 2 tablespoons honey, or 170 milliliters vegetable glycerin plus 70 milliliters water

Directions: Grind herbs into a coarse powder and put in a glass jar.

Add brandy or vodka, or vegetable glycerin and water. Stir well. If you need to add more liquid, put in an additional 30 milliliters brandy or vodka, or 25 milliliters glycerin and 5 milliliters water. Cover with a lid and let sit for 2 weeks, shaking daily.

Strain and pour liquid into a dark bottle, label, and store in a cabinet. Compost herbs. To use, take 1 teaspoon brandy or vodka elixir or 2 teaspoons glycerin elixir every day.

Tieraona Low Dog is an expert in integrative medicine, herbalist, midwife and author of Healthy at Home. *Follow her on Twitter @LowDogMD.*

Copaiba Oil:
On the Cutting Edge of Science

Discover the latest medical research on this emerging botanical remedy from the Amazon rainforest.

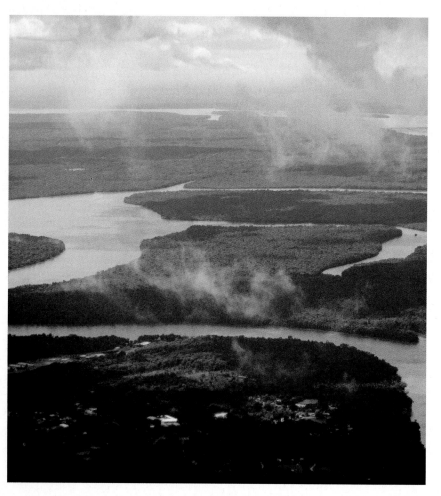

By Michelle Schoffro Cook

The vast jungle of the Amazon rainforest ensconces some of the greatest biodiversity on the planet with its 1,300 species of birds; 3,000 species of freshwater fish; and an astonishing 40,000 species of plants. It's no wonder that some of the most potent botanical remedies originate from this incredibly rich ecosystem. Among these species grows the copaiba (pronounced co-pie-EE-ba) tree (*Copaifera* spp.), towering up to 100 feet tall into the rainforest canopy. Resin extracted from the copaiba tree has only recently caught the attention of Western scientists, but it's quickly becoming one of the greatest medicinal discoveries of the plant world.

Hope for Parkinson's & Alzheimer's Diseases

Because of copaiba's interaction with the nervous system through the endocannabinoid system, it may hold the potential to counteract neurodegenerative diseases such as Parkinson's and Alzheimer's. Parkinson's disease results from a perpetual death of the dopamine neurons in the brain; but a preliminary study published in *Biomedicine & Pharmacotherapy* medical journal found that copaiba's beta-caryophyllene (BCP) interactions with the CB2 receptors might help protect and restore brain and nerve cells involved with the production and regulation of dopamine. With copaiba's ability to shield dopamine from destruction, it may hold the key to hindering the progression of Parkinson's disease.

A 2017 study published in *Evidence-Based Complementary and Alternative Medicine* explored the effects of copaiba on brain cells affected by Alzheimer's disease, in which researchers found that copaiba provided significant antioxidant, anti-inflammatory, and neuroprotective properties. Researchers also found that copaiba prevented the destruction of the brain hormone acetylcholine, a deficiency of which has been heavily linked to Alzheimer's disease.

> "In the last several years, a growing body of researchers has revived the study of copaiba and revealed what the indigenous people of the Amazon have known for centuries: Copaiba has widespread health benefits."

For the healers of the indigenous Amazon tribes, copaiba oil is nothing new. They've long used it mixed with honey to ease sore throats and tonsillitis, as well as to treat topical pain and wounds; as an antiseptic to kill bacteria in urinary tract and respiratory infections; and as an antibacterial remedy to treat bronchitis and tuberculosis. In addition, they've utilized the copaiba resin to heal stomach ulcers, syphilis, tetanus, and a variety of other afflictions.

Copaiba resin was first recorded in European medicine in 1625, after early Jesuit travelers brought it back from the New World under the name "Jesuit's Balsam." Throughout the early 1800s, doctor R. La Roche praised copaiba in medical journals, particularly for its potential cure in a case of bronchitis. In the 200 years since his findings, almost no mention of copaiba appeared in medical journals again. In the last several years, though, a growing body of researchers has revived the study of copaiba and revealed what the indigenous people have known for centuries: Copaiba has widespread health benefits.

Unlocking the Endocannabinoid System

Recent research reveals copaiba's effectiveness in relieving pain, reducing inflammation, killing germs and bacteria, inhibiting tumor growth, protecting the gastrointestinal tract, acting as a mild laxative, suppressing coughs, and expelling phlegm. According to extensive research compiled in Leslie Taylor's book, *The Healing Power of Rainforest Herbs*, copaiba supports a healthy cardiovascular, immune, digestive, nervous, and respiratory system, and acts as an antioxidant that helps destroy harmful disease-causing free radicals.

The main reason for copaiba's many health benefits stems from its ability to interact with the body's powerful endocannabinoid system (ECS). Most people aren't familiar with this recently discovered body system, as it's only been studied in-depth within the last decade.

If you've heard of cannabis, you're already somewhat familiar with the ECS; it's the same system that allows the active compounds in cannabis—

Copaiba & Cancer

Although research into the effects of copaiba on cancer is in its early stages, the oil has already shown great potential to fight cancers, given its supportive effects on the immune system. In a study published in the *European Journal of Pharmaceutical Sciences*, researchers found that copaiba stops skin cancer cells from proliferating. Researchers also found that copaiba interfered with the division of colon cancer cells, thereby reducing their ability to multiply. Authors of this study, published in *Biomedical Pharmacotherapy*, concluded that copaiba may play a role in the suppression of colon cancer, attributing these benefits—at least in part—to copaiba's anti-inflammatory properties. Copaiba may be beneficial in treating other types of cancers, including melanoma, lung, lymph, and breast cancers, but studies of copaiba's effects on these cancers are still in the preliminary phases.

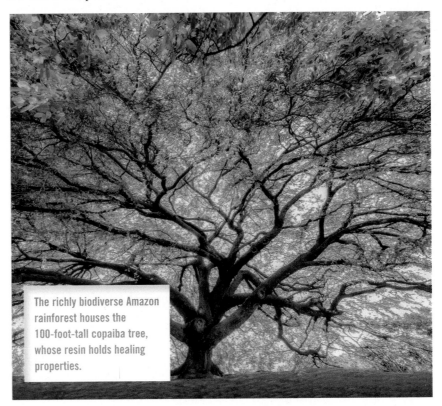

The richly biodiverse Amazon rainforest houses the 100-foot-tall copaiba tree, whose resin holds healing properties.

Antibacterial Benefits

The medical journal *Phytopherapy Research* reports that copaiba demonstrates notable antibacterial properties. The study assessed the effectiveness of various copaiba species, and found that they all had significant antibacterial activity, particularly against bacteria responsible for dental and gum conditions in the mouth. Further research found that copaiba was effective against bacterial strains such as Staphylococcus, including Methicillin-resistant Staphylococcus aureus (MRSA). This is particularly hopeful news.

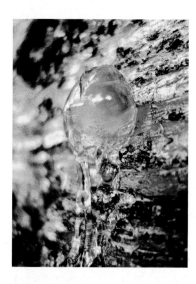

Healing Damaged Skin

Copaiba has demonstrated effectiveness against skin cancer in some studies, and other research found that the internal or topical application of copaiba oil provided significant improvement in the symptoms of chronic psoriasis by reducing scaly or thick skin. Additional research found that copaiba stimulated collagen in the skin, and promoted new skin growth, which may be beneficial for chronic wounds, burns, or the appearance of aging skin.

the cannabinoids—to interact within the body via cannabinoid receptors on cells. Since discovering these receptors throughout different parts of the body, scientists have determined that there's a network through which all of these receptors and cannabinoids interface. We can think of the ECS as a nexus between the body and mind. Growing research into the ECS opens up a world of possibility for using this network of cell receptors to combat a wide range of diseases, including neuropathic pain, mood and anxiety disorders, movement disorders such as Parkinson's and Huntington's disease, multiple sclerosis, spinal cord injuries, cancer, atherosclerosis, heart attacks, stroke, hypertension, glaucoma, metabolic syndrome, and osteoporosis.

> "Choose a sustainable product in which the company taps the trees, similarly to the way maple trees are tapped for syrup, to ensure the life and safety of the trees and ecosystem."

There are two types of cannabinoid receptors that work in tandem to regulate a diverse number of functions in the body: CB1 receptors work in the brain and nervous system, while CB2 receptors primarily function in the digestive tract and immune system. Together they modulate pain, appetite, nausea, memory, cognitive functioning, and the brain's reward center. They also work to regulate the immune system, and glandular and hormonal functions.

Three main cannabinoids interact with CB1 and CB2 receptors: tetrahydrocannabinol (THC), cannabidiol (CBD), and beta-caryophyllene (BCP). As an example, THC, the main psychoactive ingredient in cannabis, is received and processed by CB1 receptors in the brain, resulting in feelings of elation. Alternately, CBD and BCP, present in many other

plant species, have potent effects on the body through the same ECS network for a host of healing potentials. Copaiba contains high concentrations of BCP, which works exclusively on the CB2 receptors, making it particularly effective for treating digestive and immune system disorders, specifically for the reduction of hyperinflammation that results from damaged or diseased nerves.

Choosing and Using Copaiba Oil

Make sure you select high quality, pure, undiluted essential oils whenever you choose to use them for personal health. While you should always dilute essential oils in a quality carrier oil prior to full treatment, it's important to note that many oils on the market are diluted with less-than-desirable carrier oils. High-quality oils cost more than the cheap varieties on the market, but they're worth the increased price, as many cheap oils are adulterated with solvents used during the extraction process, or toxic pesticides used in growing the herbs from which essential oils are extracted.

Some companies may cut down copaiba trees to extract the oil, thereby potentially destroying the delicate rainforest. Choose a sustainable product in which the company taps the trees, similarly to the way maple trees are tapped for syrup, to ensure the life and safety of the trees and ecosystem. After diluting a drop or two in a small amount of carrier oil, always conduct a 48-hour test on a small, inconspicuous part of your skin to determine whether you have any sensitivity to the oil. Discontinue use if you experience any skin sensitivity. Use essential oils with caution and the advice of a qualified natural health practitioner during pregnancy or in the treatment of any health condition.

Once you've chosen your copaiba oil, and have tested it for any allergic reactions, you can safely begin to reap its multiple benefits. There are many ways to use copaiba essential oil: Diffuse it or mix it with water to form an aerosol for inhalation to improve your mood, or apply it topically on painful, wounded, or cancerous areas.

The Future of Copaiba

While the extent of copaiba's treatments for disease remain to be proven in scientific studies, the early findings in medical research of copaiba oil offer abounding optimism for the future of medicine. Hopefully copaiba's healing properties will continue to propel scientific research onward and fortify conclusions about its efficacy.

With more research comes the possibility for more insights into safe dosing and approved methods of application in addressing bacterial infections and disease. A more specific understanding of copaiba oil's interaction with the ECS could help treat disorders of the immune system and neurodegenerative diseases. Copaiba also holds inspiration for greater research into the possibility of treating and preventing cancer.

We have the Amazon rainforest to thank for this amazing tree and its essential oil, which, for now, can provide an alternative way to topically address pain, inflammation, and skin disorders. ❧

Michelle Schoffro Cook, PhD, DNM is an internationally best-selling and 20-time book author whose works include *Be Your Own Herbalist* and *The Cultured Cook*. Both books are available at MotherEarthNews. com/Store. Learn more about her work at FoodHouseProject.com and DrMichelleCook.com.

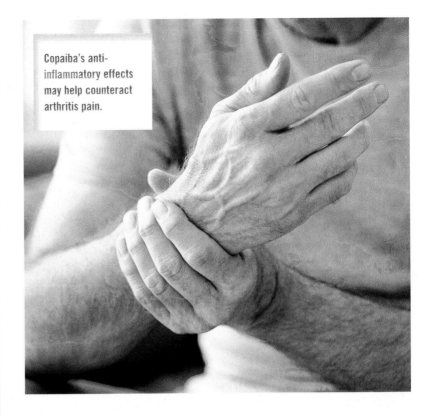

Copaiba's anti-inflammatory effects may help counteract arthritis pain.

Pain Relief for Arthritis

Some scientific studies have highlighted copaiba's anti-inflammatory effects to counteract arthritis pain. In a study published in *Complementary Therapy in Clinical Practice*, participants who received hand massages with copaiba mixed with a blend of oils known as "Deep Blue" reported 50 percent less pain, improved strength in their fingers, and increased dexterity when compared to those treated with a coconut oil placebo.

Copaiba can potentially be helpful in the treatment of arthritis and joint pain in animals, too. An animal study published in the *Journal of Cellular Biochemistry* found that copaiba demonstrated potent anti-inflammatory activity throughout the body, and reduced the number of free radicals involved in the degradation of joints in arthritic conditions. Melissa Shelton, doctor of veterinary medicine, recommends administering one drop of ingestible copaiba oil per 50 pounds, twice daily for animals. You can also apply a drop or two of the oil topically, diluted in a small amount of carrier oil.

OUR STORE

Be Your Own Herbalist
Essential Herbs for Health, Beauty, and Cooking

In *Be Your Own Herbalist*, author Michelle Schoffro Cook profiles 31 common and readily available herbs, sharing scientific discoveries about their usefulness and offering practical ways of incorporating these "Mother Nature Medicines" back into daily life.

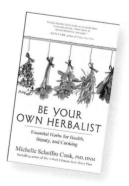

This title is available at MotherEarthNews.com/Store or by calling 800-234-3368. Mention promo code MMEPAKZ5. Item #7877.

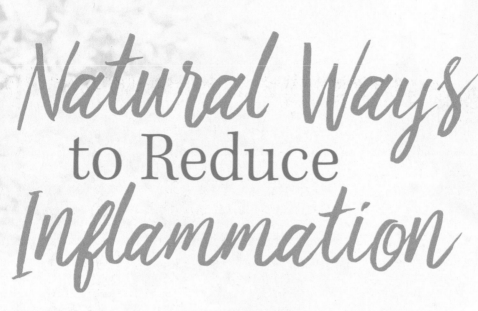

Natural Ways to Reduce Inflammation

Use these diet and lifestyle tips to ease chronic inflammation and reduce your risk of everything from cardiovascular disease to cancer.

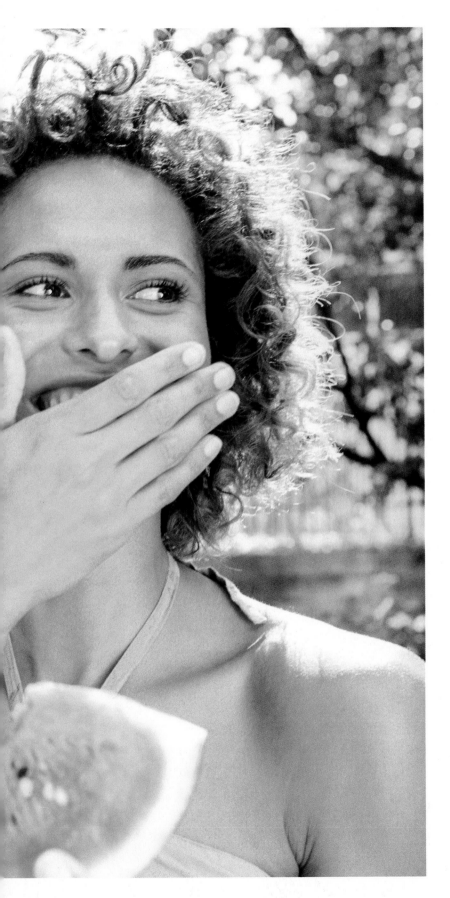

By Valerie Latona

When TV host and nutritionist Julie Daniluk developed ulcerative colitis—inflammation of the large intestine—several years ago, it ravaged her body. She not only developed severe digestive problems, she also had debilitating muscle and joint pain. But it wasn't medication that ended up curing her disease; it was a healthy, nutrient-rich diet. "After one and a half years, I'm completely in remission," Daniluk says. "If I can come back from this disease and be 100 percent healthy, imagine what you can do if you don't have a serious health problem like this. We can do so much to shift the course of our health by just eating an anti-inflammatory diet."

But what's all the fuss about inflammation, a so-called health bad guy that seems to gain more notoriety with every passing year? Despite its bad reputation, not all inflammation is bad; in fact, inflammation is the core of our body's healing—and immune—response. When something harmful or irritating affects a part of our body, an inflammatory cascade of events is set in motion: Blood flow increases to that area, and along with it healing proteins and infection-fighting white blood cells. Without inflammation, wounds and infections would never heal.

As with stress, though, some inflammation is healthy, but chronic inflammation—which some experts describe as an immune system response that's out of control—is not.

"Inflammation is a form of cellular and chemical warfare in the body," says David L. Katz, director of the Yale-Griffin Prevention Research Center in Derby, Connecticut, and author of *Disease-Proof*. "But as with all warfare, there is potential for collateral damage. Chronic inflammation stresses and injures cells, causing them to malfunction and age." This malfunctioning, in turn, can trigger disease. Study after study suggests that everything from cardiovascular disease and cancer to joint issues and even skin problems like psoriasis can be the result of unchecked inflammation in the body.

What Causes Inflammation?

This list includes the biggest triggers of chronic inflammation in the body.

Just as there are plenty of ways to trigger the body's inflammatory cascade, there are plenty of ways we can ease chronic inflammation. "The same six lifestyle factors exert the greatest influence on all major chronic disease risk factors," researcher David L. Katz says. "These are feet (physical activity), forks (a healthy diet), fingers (don't smoke), sleep (get enough), stress (learn to manage it), and love (cultivate loving relationships)." But most experts agree that, when it comes to inflammation, food is the first, and most important, place to start.

■ **Sugar and processed foods, particularly those with unhealthy trans fats:** "White sugar is the most inflammatory substance on the planet," says nutritionist Julie Daniluk, who adds that anything that causes a fast spike in blood sugar levels such as white flour triggers an inflammatory response. Eat them regularly, and we're keeping our inflammation levels on overdrive. Better sweetener bets include stevia and coconut sugar, which don't raise blood sugar levels like processed sugar does. Raw honey and maple syrup are also good options.

■ **Genetically modified (GMO) foods:** There's a reason so many health experts are speaking out against GMOs. "Any food modified from its original self is no longer the same food," says Jeffrey Morrison, a doctor and author of *Cleanse Your Body, Clear Your Mind*. While to date no formal research has studied the effect of GMO foods on humans, in vivo studies have shown that when a body encounters a GMO food (or any food that doesn't "agree" with us, Morrison says), it doesn't recognize it and tries to protect us from it with symptoms of inflammation (this could range from bloating and digestive upset to gas and pain). Ignore our bodies' red flags and, over time, the inflammation could become chronic.

■ **Chemicals in our environment:** "From pesticides to parabens, chemicals in our environment have a strong estrogenic effect on our bodies," Morrison says. "Too many estrogens can cause an inflammatory state." To avoid as many environmental chemicals as possible, Morrison recommends eating organic fruits and vegetables whenever you can; avoiding plastics, which can contain the endocrine disruptor bisphenol-A (BPA) and other estrogenic chemicals; and avoiding food in cans

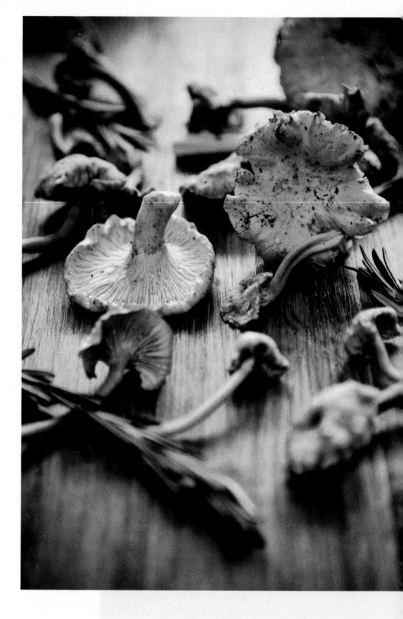

lined with BPA. A few brands such as Eden Organic (EdenFoods.com) offer BPA-free cans; otherwise choose fresh food or food packed in glass jars.

■ **Heavy metals:** Mercury (from fatty fish such as swordfish and tuna) and lead are heavy metals that are toxic to the body and can fuel inflammation. "Heavy metals essentially cause our bodies to rust because of oxidative stress—the same mechanism that causes rust to form on metal," Morrison says. To find out if your levels are high, have your doctor order a whole-blood mercury test and a lead test, two separate blood tests typically covered by insurance. Then stick to lower-mercury seafood sources such as wild salmon, tilapia, clams, and mussels.

Eat to Beat Inflammation

Research finds that the more sugar, red meat, processed meat, fried foods, and dairy people eat, the higher their indicators of inflammation. In one study, researchers at Icahn School of Medicine at Mount Sinai in New York City found that fried and processed foods can increase inflammation, while cutting back on these foods can "restore the body's natural defenses." In a study published in the *Journal of the American College of Cardiology*, Greek researchers found that those who eat a plant-based, healthy-fat Mediterranean diet (heavy on produce but light on meat, white flour, and white sugar) have lower inflammation levels. The reason: The right nutrients seem to guard against inflammation, and some even help to calm inflammation already present. Try this list of some of the best inflammation-fighting foods around.

■ **Amaranth:** "Amaranth is a seed that acts like a grain," says holistic health coach Kristine Nicholson, a healthy eating specialist for Whole Foods Market in Millburn, New Jersey. "But it's got a whole lot more nutrition than grains." It contains about four times as much calcium as wheat, and twice as much iron and magnesium. Plus, it's gluten-free and easy to digest — a good option for those with food sensitivities or allergies. Other best bets: quinoa, millet, and wild rice, which is lower in carbs and higher in protein than brown rice.

■ **Ginger:** "Ginger belongs to a class of herbs called bitter herbs," says Jeffrey Morrison, a New York City-based doctor and author of *Cleanse Your Body, Clear Your Mind.* "Horseradish is another one. They're very good anti-inflammatories." Ginger—which contains potent anti-inflammatory compounds called gingerols—helps prevent the body from manufacturing prostaglandins and leukotrienes, both of which trigger inflammation. Studies have found ginger extract reduces the swelling and pain associated with osteoarthritis and rheumatoid arthritis. Drink ginger tea and use fresh ginger in everything from soups to stir-fries.

■ **Grass-Fed Beef:** Conventionally raised red meat contains unhealthy ratios of omega-6 to omega-3, as high as 20:1, which is why it's considered bad for the heart and just about every other organ in the body. But organic grass-fed red meat is rich in inflammation-quelling omega-3 fatty acids, and has a ratio of omega-6s to omega-3s around the ideal 4:1. It's also rich in B vitamins, selenium, and zinc. Daniluk, author of *Meats that Heal Inflammation*, suggests mixing up the kind of grass-fed meat you eat; try bison, elk, and venison, too. But never chargrill meats. This creates advanced glycation end products, which promote inflammation by damaging essential proteins.

■ **Green Tea:** Numerous studies prove the anti-inflammatory benefits of green tea, made from unfermented leaves. The reason? Green tea contains one of the highest concentrations of powerful antioxidants called catechins, including potent epigallocatechin gallate, or EGCG. One study found that EGCG might block the overproduction of pro-

> "Those who eat a plant-based, healthy-fat Mediterranean diet (heavy on produce but light on meat, white flour, and white sugar) have lower inflammation levels."

inflammatory substances. Other studies have linked tea drinking (at least two cups per day) to a reduced risk of heart disease and stroke, lower cholesterol levels, and even lower rates of cancer. "Drink organic, whole-leaf green tea to get the full benefits," Nicholson says.

■ **Kale:** Bitter vegetables such as kale, spinach, radishes, broccoli raab, and mustard greens have anti-inflammatory effects because of their high antioxidant levels. But all brightly colored fruits and vegetables—from blueberries to red bell peppers—are rich in inflammation-quelling antioxidants, too. These compounds help neutralize the harmful free radicals that trigger inflammation and disease.

■ **Mushrooms:** Mushrooms are the only vegetable source of vitamin D—a hormone that plays a key role in immune system health—if they've grown under ultraviolet (UV) light. (Like humans, mushrooms produce vitamin D when exposed to UV light.) One study in *The Journal of Immunology* found that vitamin D is key for inhibiting the inflammatory cascade in the body, particularly in people with chronic inflammatory diseases such as asthma, arthritis, and prostate cancer. You typically get 400 IU of vitamin D per 1 cup of mushrooms.

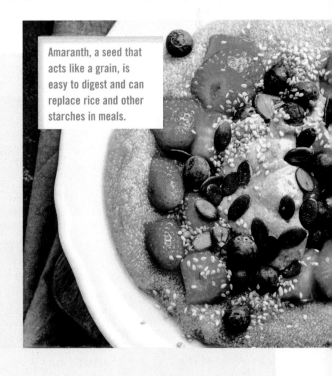

Amaranth, a seed that acts like a grain, is easy to digest and can replace rice and other starches in meals.

4 Daily Tweaks That Reduce Inflammation

A healthy diet goes a long way, but add in these simple everyday changes and you can help get inflammation under control for years to come.

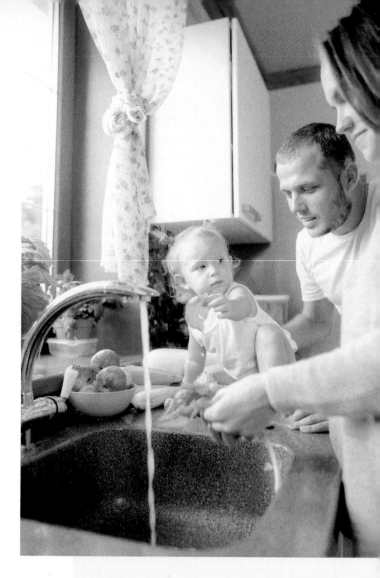

■ **Get more sleep:** Scientists at Emory University School of Medicine in Atlanta found that sleep deprivation or poor sleep quality raises inflammation in the body. "Sleep—at least seven and a half to eight hours a night—is extremely useful for recharging the body and decreasing inflammatory hormones like cortisol and adrenaline," says doctor Jeffrey Morrison, author of *Cleanse Your Body, Clear Your Mind*. "It's these stress hormones that make the body more susceptible to inflammation." Finding it hard to sleep at night? Don't use electronic devices (including TV, computer, or your smartphone) for at least two hours before going to bed. Studies have shown that the blue light emitted by these devices can interfere with the production of a key sleep hormone, melatonin. Also, shut off your Wi-Fi before you go to bed; some experts believe the signals can interfere with our bodies' own electrical impulses during the night, making us more agitated or anxious and unable to sleep soundly.

■ **Exercise regularly:** A University of Illinois study found that exercise seems to help heal chronic inflammation in the skin—a benefit that could be extrapolated to the entire body, the researchers say. The study, published in the *American Journal of Physiology*, found that exercise helps increase blood flow in the body and decreases the amount of inflammatory molecules released in the body. Another study conducted by Mark Hamer, an epidemiologist at University College London, found that just two and a half hours of moderate exercise per week (about 20 minutes a day) reduced markers of inflammation by 12 percent.

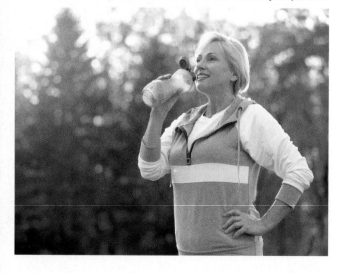

The reason? When we exercise, our fat and muscle tissues release bursts of proteins called cytokines into our bloodstream, helping inflammation to drop.

■ **Maintain a healthy weight:** Fat causes inflammation, says New Jersey-based integrative doctor Kristine Gedroic. "Your fat is not the product of your inflammation; it becomes the source of your inflammation." For good health, we must keep our weight within a healthy range. Excess weight around the middle, particularly, is an active source of hormones and inflammatory compounds. When we lose excess weight, our bodies' inflammation levels decrease. One study at the Fred Hutchinson Cancer Research Center in Seattle found that when overweight or obese women dropped at least 5 percent of their body weight, they had measurable declines in markers of inflammation.

■ **Reduce stress:** Chronically high levels of stress hormones can lead to the release of excess inflammatory chemicals. This is why finding ways to lower your stress every day (such as breathing exercises, yoga, meditation, or a daily tea ritual) is key to staying healthy.

■ **Oregano:** This herb contains an active agent called rosmarinic acid that's extremely rich in free radical-fighting antioxidants. But nearly all herbs are rich in antioxidants that can help fight inflammation. Many herbs are also antimicrobial. "Much of what we're seeing today is the presence of infections in the body that trigger inflammation," says Kristine Gedroic, an integrative family practitioner based in Morristown, New Jersey, pointing to research on bacteria-triggered gum disease linked to inflammatory conditions such as arthritis and Alzheimer's disease. Skip the spice jars, though. Fresh is best when it comes to herbs. "Have your own herb garden—on your windowsill or in your backyard," Gedroic says. "It truly is nature's pharmacy." (Learn how at MotherEarthNews.com/Grow-Herbs.)

■ **Organic Coconut Kefir:** Dairy tops many pro-inflammatory food lists, which is why many experts recommend dairy-free alternatives. Coconut-based kefir (made by fermenting coconut milk), yogurt-style cultured coconut milk, and fermented coconut water are all rich in live probiotics, healthy bacteria that displace bad bacteria in the gut. "Seventy percent of the immune system is in the digestive tract," Morrison says. "Healthy bacteria, or probiotics, help regulate the immune system, thereby helping reduce inflammation." Make sure the label says "live and active cultures."

■ **Turmeric:** This potent anti-inflammatory seems to inhibit eicosanoids, molecules that play a key role in the inflammatory response. One study found that supplements of curcumin (turmeric's active ingredient) reduced levels of C-reactive protein, a general inflammation marker linked to arthritis and cardiovascular disease. Another study of people with early-stage Alzheimer's disease found that curcumin seems to inhibit formation of the inflammatory plaque that accompanies the disease. Look for organic turmeric root; make tea or add it to eggs, salad dressings, and vegetable dishes. Or take supplements: Integrative doctor Andrew Weil recommends 400 to 600 mg of standardized 95 percent curcuminoids, three times a day for patients with arthritis, tendonitis, and autoimmune disorders. Avoid it if you have gallstones, bile duct dysfunction, or are pregnant.

Bottom line when it comes to an anti-inflammatory diet: "Eating healthy is eating anti-inflammatory," Nicholson says. When we eat the most nutrient-rich foods we can at every meal, over time we shed excess weight, have more energy, and feel healthier overall—all while reducing our risk of inflammation-driven disease. "When we take out inflammatory foods and put into our bodies anti-inflammatory nutrition, then we start to experience a profound shift," Daniluk says. "You can quickly lose your appetite for foods that can cause inflammation." 🌱

Valerie Latona is the former editor-in-chief of *Shape*. She is also a health writer and the founder of ValerieLatona.com, a healthy living website. A passionate advocate of healthy living, Latona lives in New Jersey with her husband and three young children.

Kale with Honeyed Macadamia Nuts

Bitter vegetables like kale have an anti-inflammatory effect because of their high antioxidant levels. Try this new take on kale from Whole Foods Market's Kristine Nicholson. **Serves 6.**

Ingredients
- 2 tablespoons honey, divided
- ½ cup roasted and salted macadamia nuts
- 2 bunches kale, thick stems removed, leaves thinly sliced
- 2 tablespoons white wine vinegar
- 1½ tablespoons creamy almond butter

Directions: Preheat oven to 350 F. In a medium bowl, toss 1 tablespoon honey with nuts and 1 teaspoon water.

Bake on a parchment-paper-lined baking sheet, tossing 2 or 3 times, until golden brown (about 10 to 12 minutes). Cool, and roughly chop. Set aside.

Arrange kale in a large, deep skillet.

In a medium bowl, whisk together vinegar, almond butter, remaining honey, and 2 tablespoons of water. Drizzle over kale, cover, and cook over medium heat, tossing occasionally until wilted and just tender (about 5 minutes). Scatter nuts over top, and serve.

Kristine Nicholson

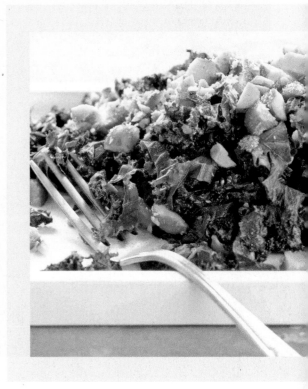

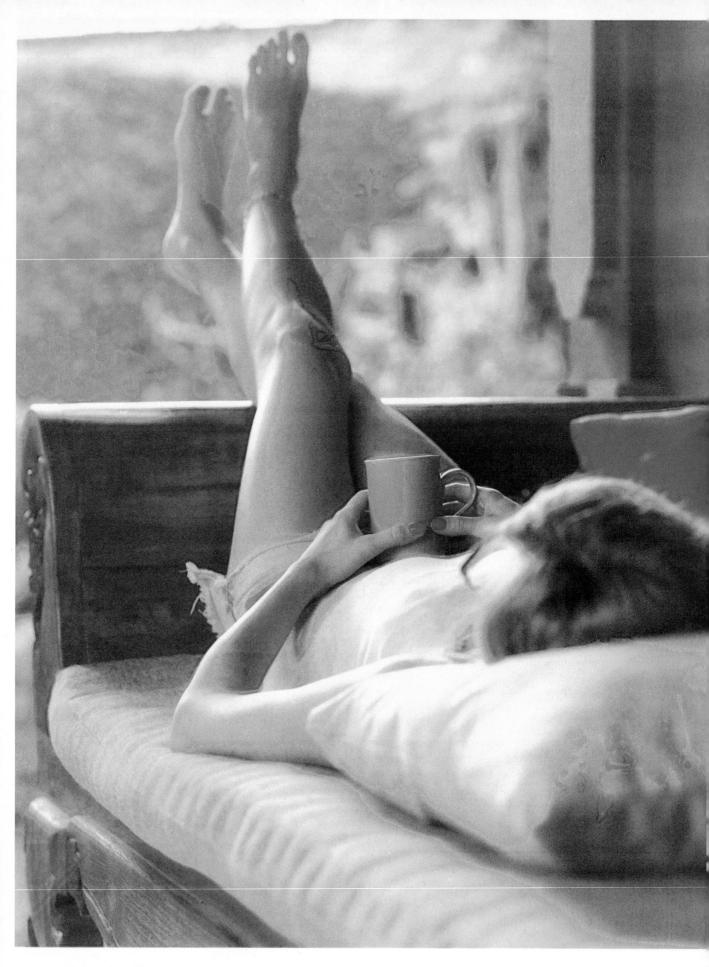

Old-Time Herbal Remedies to Relieve Stress

Uncover age-old herbal remedies to relieve stress in your daily life.

By Sharon L. Hagemann

Whether you're struggling to get the harvest in before the first frost or you're stuck in a rush-hour traffic jam, stress has become a fact of life for many of us these days. We get worn to a frazzle by work demands or pushed to our limits by family needs. Nearly everyone feels overwhelmed at one point or another, and most of us aren't even aware of the sources of stress in our lives or how our bodies attempt to cope. Over time, however, the effects of stress can pose a serious challenge to our emotional, mental, and physical well-being.

Research into the physiological effects of stress has revealed a series of reactions known collectively as the General Adaptation Syndrome. Alarm reaction, the response that first occurs when you're faced with a perceived emotional or physical threat, results in a rise in blood pressure, an increased heartbeat, and a general mobilization of your body's defensive forces.

The alarm reaction stage is followed by the resistance stage, which comes when you've adapted to the threat and your symptoms—sweaty palms, clenched jaw—begin to improve or disappear. Luckily, most physical and emotional stress situations are contained within these two stages. However, a third response, known as the exhaustion stage, will set in if you regularly feel anxious over a prolonged period of time. A constant battle with stress will cause alarm reaction symptoms to reappear. If the stress continues unabated, health problems such as hypertension, chronic anxiety, and even heart attack can ensue. Use these herbal remedies to relieve stress from work and life.

Mountains Out of Molehills

An obvious and daunting fact about stress is that it has less to do with external factors (your car breaking down, your kids bickering) than with your very conscious reaction to these events. In other words, we are in charge of our own stress levels.

Different situations trigger stress in different people. For instance, your co-worker might cringe at the thought of giving a lecture in front of a large audience, while you might jump at the chance. Likewise, one person will relish an active schedule full of challenges, while another will prefer quieter, more predictable pursuits. Switch these two types of people and each would feel stressed in the other one's shoes.

Another fact we often overlook is that stress can come from good occasions as well as bad ones. Even happy events such as a wedding, a promotion, or the birth of a new baby can prove stressful. The anticipation and excitement of added responsibility that comes with positive growth and change can cause just as many migraine headaches and stomach jitters as a bad event such as a tax audit. Again, the way the situation affects your health and well-being depends largely on how you react.

Modify your responses to life's events and you'll feel more calm and in control, even though applying the brakes, taking a deep breath, and getting centered as the rest of the world accelerates is much easier said than done. With a little practice, though, you can do it—and you'll appreciate your newfound sense of calm the next time you're faced with a crisis. Try these simple, everyday stress-reducing habits I've included here (see Page 88). I recommend these tips to patients who find their lives getting out of control. If these tips work well for you, you might consider deepening your relaxation response by using mind-body techniques such as yoga and meditation.

Herbal treatments can also help balance body and soul. Some of these plants target physical ailments, while others address psychological concerns. For example, if you are under extreme pressure, your heart races and you feel short of breath, you might find relief in motherwort, a natural tranquilizer. If stress ties you in knots and nauseates you, try fennel or lemon balm. Tense, sore muscles generally respond favorably to cramp bark. Feverfew and willow bark work well for migraine and tension

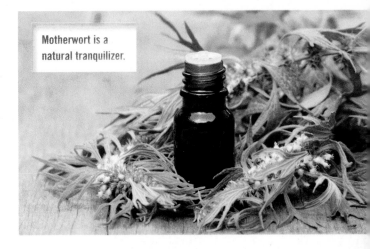

Motherwort is a natural tranquilizer.

9 Stress-Free Habits

■ **Love, Laugh, Let Go:** Putting too much pressure on yourself only creates more tension. Don't judge yourself too harshly, or expect more of yourself than you expect of others. Instead, accept yourself and your faults. Research demonstrates that those who take things in stride have higher self-esteem and less stress, which translates into better health.

■ **Create Your Own Rituals:** Savor a cup of chamomile tea in the late afternoon. Light some jasmine incense and a candle during bathtime. Making space in your schedule for simple rituals can go a long way in easing stress. No matter how hectic life may be, you'll find comfort in knowing that at least some things remain sacred.

■ **Get Silly:** Laughter increases blood flow to the brain, raises endorphin levels, and lowers levels of stress hormones. Plus, doing it just feels great. When you're feeling down, call up a friend who never fails to make you laugh. It really is the best medicine.

■ **Reap Your Rewards:** Rewards for your hard work needn't be expensive—just something pleasurable to look forward to. Buy yourself some flowers, take a garden stroll at the end of a long day, or celebrate your job promotion at the ice cream parlor with friends.

■ **Make Time for Meals:** Eating at your desk or on-the-go is a ready-made recipe for heartburn and mental fatigue. Take time out to nourish and replenish your body, no matter how long your to-do list might be that day.

■ **Learn From Children:** "Take five" and watch some small children at play. They're enjoying the moment and aren't worried about the past or future. Try following their example.

■ **Find a Hobby:** Do something purely for the fun of it. Gather coins from foreign lands, make scented candles, or put on a pair of cross-country skis and see where they take you. Indulge in something that makes your heart sing.

■ **Set Priorities:** Devote some time to think about your life goals. List your goals for the year, the week, and the day. This should give you a good idea of what you are really seeking. Always go after the important things first, and be open to the fact that your goals may evolve over time.

■ **Write it Down:** Putting pen to paper can be healthy and cathartic; reading over what you have written often helps put things into perspective. If stress has you losing sleep, jot down your worries in a notebook before going to bed. Let them go, and you won't feel the need to process them all night in your head.

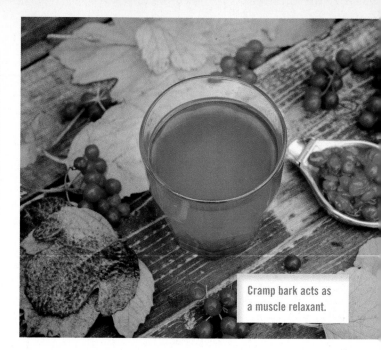

Cramp bark acts as a muscle relaxant.

headaches. If it's sleep that's eluding you, passionflower or skullcap might just do the trick. And should you find yourself stressed out and depressed, reach for St. John's wort, a natural antidepressant.

The following, in a nutshell, is information on some popular and effective herbal remedies to relieve stress. Although all of these herbs are safe, you may wish to confer with a qualified herbalist or natural health-care provider to see which ones are best suited to your particular needs and situation. He or she may also have additional suggestions to help you deal with long-term stress in your life.

Stress-Free Herbs

Cramp Bark (*Viburnum opulus*): While commonly called "high cranberry," this plant is in no sense related to the edible cranberry, which belongs to the elder family. Cramp bark acts as a muscle relaxant, making it beneficial for elite athletes and hardworking gardeners alike.

Preparation: Recommended in extract form (40 drops, four times per day). It usually works within 30 minutes.

Fennel (*Foeniculum vulgare*): A favorite in the herbal healing arena from the time of the pharaohs to the present day, fennel gently relieves gastrointestinal upsets, flatulence, abdominal tension and colic.

Preparation: Take in capsule form (one to three times daily) or by extract (40 drops after meals). You'll notice relief from gas or nausea within half an hour of ingestion.

Note: Since, fennel has an estrogenic effect, women advised by their doctors not to take birth control pills should avoid the herb in medicinal amounts.

Feverfew (*Chrysanthemum parthenium*): This ancient herb had all but fallen out of use until the late 1970s, when scientific trials established its validity as a "modern miracle" for the relief of migraine headaches.

Preparation: Take three capsules, three times daily. Serious migraine sufferers may find it takes several months to achieve maximum effectiveness.

Note: Some people develop mouth sores and nausea using feverfew. It should also be avoided during pregnancy.

Lemon Balm (*Melissa officinalis*): Medieval Europeans used lemon balm to allay nervousness and anxiety. More recently, researchers have discovered that lemon balm oil appears to have mild tranquilizing properties, substantiating its use as a mild sedative.

Preparation: Make an infusion by steeping 2 teaspoons of the herb in 8 ounces of water in a covered container for 20 minutes. Administer up to four times per day. The effects are cumulative and should be felt after a week's worth of treatment.

Motherwort (*Leonorus cardiaca*): The ancient Greeks and Romans prescribed motherwort for both palpitations and depression. Contemporary herbalists recognize its use as a mild sedative and anxiety reducer.

Preparation: I recommend a tincture because the herb is extremely bitter. Take ½ to 1 teaspoon, twice a day (effective within a week). Severe anxiety responds best to regular use over a one-month period.

Note: Motherwort has been shown to suppress thyroid function in large doses.

Passionflower (*Passiflora incarnata*): Documented as a tranquilizer and sedative in the National Formulary from 1916 to 1936, passionflower acts as a gentle tranquilizer, pain reliever, and digestive aid.

Preparation: For a relaxing, sleep-inducing infusion, steep 1 teaspoon of leaves in a cup of boiling water for 15 minutes. Take one cup at bedtime for insomnia. For general relaxation, try sipping up to three cups a day.

Note: Passionflower is generally considered safe, although extremely large doses may cause nausea and/or vomiting in some individuals.

St. John's Wort (*Hypericum perforatum*): In the Middle Ages, legend stated that this red-resined plant sprang from the blood of John the Baptist when he was beheaded. Therefore, it was often blessed by a priest and worn around the neck to ward off disease and temptation. Today, St. John's wort is used to relieve anxiety and restore emotional stability. Its active component, hypericin, combats depression in the higher centers of the brain. It is of particular use to those with chronic anxiety, or to individuals who suffer from panic attacks.

Preparation: Take 20 to 30 drops of standardized extract, four times a day. It is a slow but enduring tranquilizer that must be used an average of 10 days before effects are noted.

Note: This herb can have photosensitizing effect for some users. Avoid exposure to sun during a course of treatment, as sunburn will quickly result. Also, contact your health-care provider before taking if you already take prescription antidepressants.

Skullcap (*Scutellaria lateriflora*): Eclectic American physicians of the 19th century recommended skullcap as a tranquilizer and sedative for insomnia and nervousness. It relieves mood swings, sleeping disorders, nervous tension, and stress-related headaches.

Preparation: Take 30 to 40 drops of fresh plant tincture in juice or tea up to four times a day. Skullcap works over a period of several weeks.

Note: While there have been no reports of toxicity, large amounts of tincture may result in confusion, twitching, and convulsions.

Willow Bark (*Salix alba*): Yet another time-tested "herbal aspirin" (in fact, the original ingredient in commercial aspirin), white willow bark is greatly effective in relieving head pain, particularly tension headaches. It also reduces fever and inflammations.

Preparation: Gently boil 2 teaspoons of herb in 8 ounces of water for 15 minutes. Remove from heat, cover, and steep for an additional 30 minutes. Take up to three cups a day, or three capsules three times a day. Willow bark's effects can generally be felt within two to three hours.

Note: Willow bark contains tannin, which can cause constipation. ❧

Sharon L. Hagemann was a freelance writer and a doctor of naturopathic medicine.

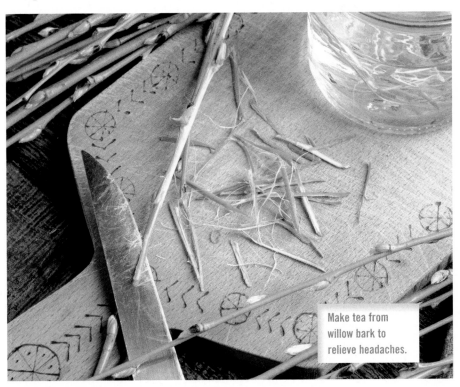

Make tea from willow bark to relieve headaches.

St. John's Wort

Get to know this sometimes controversial herb.

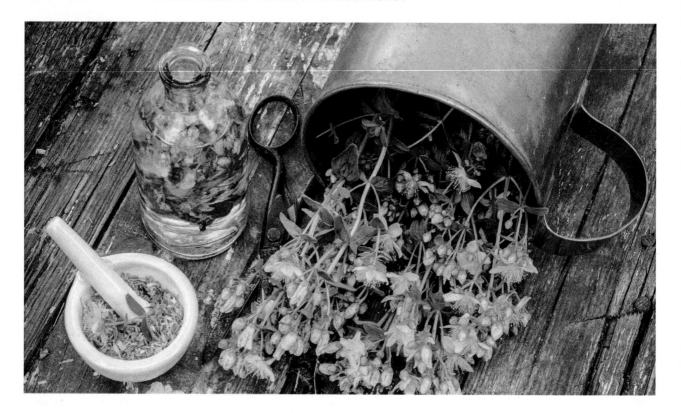

By the *Mother Earth News* editors

Some people swear by it and others swear at it. In its native Europe, St. John's wort is not a cause for complaint, but elsewhere its rampant habits and toxicity have made it planta non grata.

The genus *Hypericum* (which is variously assigned to the families Hypericaceae, Guttiferae, or Clusiaceae) contains some 300 species of plants ranging from creeping forms to 15-foot-tall shrubs. The species most familiar to herb gardeners is *H. perforatum*, found along roadsides and in fields and waste sites throughout much of North America and elsewhere. It is an erect, branching plant, growing 1 to 2½ feet tall. The stems, which may be woody at the base, bear two lengthwise ridges and are sparsely clothed with pairs of 1-inch-long narrow leaves. These leaves are dotted with translucent oil glands that look like perforations, giving rise to the species name, *perforatum*. The ends of the stems bear showy, rounded or flat-topped clusters of 1-inch-wide bright yellow flowers. The five petals are often bordered with tiny black dots and yield a reddish resinous sap when crushed. The most striking feature of this and other hypericums is the bushy clump of stamens that bursts from the center of the flower. Bees visit them for their abundant pollen, but the flowers produce no nectar, and the seeds develop without fertilization. The fruit is a three-celled capsule that opens to reveal small, shiny black resinous seeds. All parts of the plant smell like turpentine.

Many species of *Hypericum* are more ornamental, with a neater habit and showier flowers, than *H. perforatum*. One that is available in many nurseries is creeping St. John's wort (*H. calycinum*), a shrubby form with larger leaves and 2-inch bright yellow flowers that is often grown as a ground cover.

Legends

Legends about St. John's wort go back to antiquity. It was thought to ward off witches and annoying fairies as well as to protect one from thunder. Some believe that the generic name, hypericum, is derived from the Greek words *hyper* ("above") and *eikon* ("image"), referring to the custom of hanging a sprig above a picture to repel evil spirits; others hold that hypericum means "above an apparition" and refers to the power of the odor to banish spirits. A more prosaic theory is that hypericum comes from Greek words meaning "above (or below) the heather" and refers (maybe) to where the plants grow or to their relative height.

Early Christians adopted the herb as a symbol of St. John the Baptist, perhaps because it flowered on June 24, when his birth was celebrated. Some also observed that the leaves "bled" red oil on August 29, the anniversary of his beheading. (These dates may have been adjusted with the later adoption of the Gregorian calendar, but the observations still apply as plants bloom from June through September, and the leaves exude oil on crushing throughout the growing season.)

Other beliefs about the protective power of St. John's wort persisted. For example, sleeping with a piece of the herb under the pillow on St. John's Eve would ensure the saint's blessing and protection from dying during the coming year. Welsh families predicted life expectancies by hanging a sprig for each member and noting the next day how shriveled the leaves were.

Medicinal Uses

The history of St. John's wort as a medicinal herb has ancient roots. Early English herbalists esteemed it as a treatment for deep sword cuts and other wounds. According to the "doctrine of signatures," the oil glands in the leaves resembled pores in the skin, suggesting that the herb must be good for healing skin problems. The red oil extracted from the flowers by soaking them in olive or other vegetable oil was used externally to treat burns, neuralgia, hard tumors, caked breasts, bruises, and sciatica.

The herb has been taken internally to treat cancer, rabies, gout, arthritis, respiratory and gastrointestinal ailments, menstrual cramps, and nervous disorders. Reputed to be a diuretic, it also has been and continues to be prescribed to cure bedwetting.

American Indians used *H. perforatum* and other hypericums to treat a wide range of ills. For example, the Cherokee used *H. perforatum* to reduce fever, promote menstruation, and treat diarrhea, nosebleed, venereal disease, and snakebite; they washed their babies with an infusion of the roots to make them strong. The Fox and Menominee used the related *H. ascyron* in a tuberculosis remedy.

Present-day herbalists consider St. John's wort a relaxing restorative and prescribe it for insomnia, depression, and unpleasant symptoms associated with menopause. The oil is applied externally to relieve the pain of neuralgia and promote the healing of burns, bruises, and hemorrhoids, and is taken internally for intestinal disorders.

A number of studies in the past decade have suggested that St. John's wort has some antidepressant effect. Extracts of St. John's wort have been shown to inhibit the growth of the bacterium that causes tuberculosis. Other studies have confirmed anti-inflammatory, antiseptic, and antispasmodic activity. The hopes that St. John's wort might be a cure for cancer and a treatment of AIDS apparently have not been fulfilled. The principal active constituent is hypericin, the red pigment in the oil.

Despite its long history and current use in Europe as a healing herb, St. John's wort has been judged unsafe by the FDA. When the herb is taken internally, the hypericin can sensitize nerve endings to sunlight, causing dermatitis when the skin is subsequently exposed to the sun. In some individuals, this photosensitivity can be activated merely by touching the plant, as it can with rue.

Other Uses

St. John's wort doesn't hold a prominent place in the kitchen, except perhaps in arrangements of cut flowers. The tops can be made into a beverage tea that is somewhat bitter and astringent, and the flowers have been used to flavor mead (a fermented beverage that contains honey) and vermouth.

The red pigment has been used as a dyestuff for silk and wool. The flowers yield a deep violet-red dye. Using a tin mordant produces an orange-red, and an alum mordant gives yellow. The stems yield a brown dye with alum.

Growing It

St. John's wort is hardy to Zone 3 and also grows well in the South. It thrives in poor to average soil and is not particular as to soil pH. Plant it in full sun or part shade. Seeds germinate best if not covered; just press them into moist soil. Plants will spread of their own accord, or you can increase them faster by rooting stem cuttings or taking root divisions.

Not Growing It

In some parts of the world, ranchers would just as soon St. John's wort didn't increase at all. The same photosensitivity reaction following ingestion of St. John's wort mentioned above has killed or injured millions of grazing animals, particularly light-colored ones, in the western U.S., Canada, Australia, and New Zealand. St. John's wort is thus considered "one of the most toxic pasture weeds in New Zealand." It aggressively takes over rangelands, especially those that have been overgrazed.

Even though animals do not relish the herb, they eat it if they are hungry enough. Shedding of the wool or hair, swelling of the face, loss of appetite, blindness, and death from starvation may follow. Efforts to eliminate St. John's wort have included plowing it under, repeated mowing, and herbicides, but the only effective control has been the introduction of two European species of beetle whose only food plant is *H. perforatum*. While the beetles seem to keep the plants in check, they don't keep the species from spreading to new areas and driving out native species. In Colorado, St. John's wort grew for years in one restricted site, nibbled on by one of the species of beetle, but recently plants have been discovered elsewhere in the state, and St. John's wort now shows signs of becoming a major pest. ❧

The Medicinal Uses of CBD Oil

Look past the stigma that accompanies cannabis to learn the health benefits of hemp-derived cannabidiol oil.

By Lydia Noyes

Ask 10 people today about their thoughts on cannabis, and then prepare to listen to 10 different answers. Despite being part of a national dialogue for decades, the controversy over this plant still leaves many of us with more questions than answers.

Hemp-derived cannabidiol (CBD) oil is an increasingly prevalent ingredient in supplements and wellness products on the market, but there's plenty of confusion about what this compound really is. How is CBD connected to marijuana, and will it improve your health? Most importantly, is it legal?

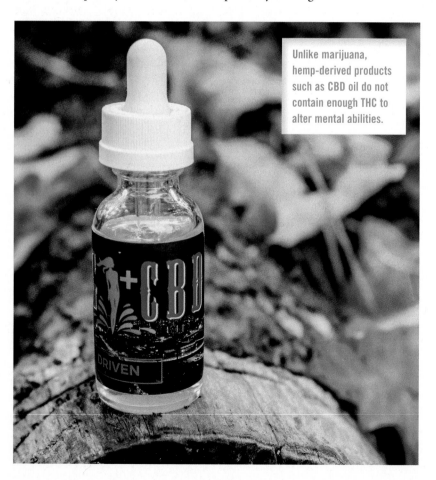

Unlike marijuana, hemp-derived products such as CBD oil do not contain enough THC to alter mental abilities.

What is CBD Oil?

One of humanity's oldest crops, hemp (*Cannabis sativa*) was first cultivated as a textile fiber around 8000 B.C. in Iran and Iraq. Part of the plant's appeal is how easy it is to grow, as hemp requires little water and few (if any) pesticides. Today, it's raised on an industrial scale and used for manufacturing biofuels, health foods, organic body-care products, and plastic composites.

Contrary to popular opinion, hemp and marijuana aren't the same. While both originate from *Cannabis sativa*, centuries of selective breeding have produced dramatically different crops. To be considered marijuana, a cannabis plant must contain at least 0.3 percent of the mind-altering tetrahydrocannabinol (THC) compound. More typically, marijuana contains a THC concentration of 5 to 30 percent. In contrast, hemp plants legally must contain 0.3 percent THC or less, and it is from hemp that most CBD oil is derived.

THC and CBD are two of the more than 70 named chemical compounds found in cannabis that — along with other more obscure compounds — are collectively known as cannabinoids. CBD alone can constitute up to 40 percent of hemp plant extracts. Specialized extraction methods can pull a pure or highly concentrated form of CBD oil that's rich in omega-3 fatty acids, amino acids, terpenes, antioxidants,

0.3%

The maximum amount of THC a *Cannabis sativa* plant can contain to legally be labeled "hemp."

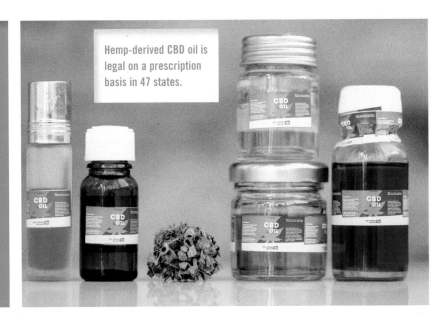

Hemp-derived CBD oil is legal on a prescription basis in 47 states.

and other beneficial compounds. For this reason, CBD oil is often taken orally through nutritional supplements, capsules, and even chewing gum, and it has also developed into a variety of wellness products that allow it to be absorbed through the skin.

THC, CBD, and the Role of Cannabinoids

How did CBD oil earn its reputation as a wonder product for health? The secret lies in the cannabinoids. These chemical compounds are naturally found in your body's endocannabinoid system (ECS) and are consumed as phytocannabinoids through plants we eat such as flax, chocolate, and carrots. These compounds help manage regulatory processes, including sleep cycle, mood, and appetite.

Different cannabinoids work by attaching themselves to either CB1 or CB2 receptors in your body. THC attaches specifically to CB1 receptors, which control coordination, movement, mood, cognition, appetite, and memory formation. This explains why it alters consciousness and produces a chemical high.

In contrast, CBD affects CB2 receptors, which are predominantly involved in regulating pain and

inflammation throughout the immune system. While it was once thought that CBD targeted these receptors directly, the consensus today is that the compound triggers the body to create its own cannabinoids that attach there instead. Regardless, the result is the same: CBD works to reduce physical pain and inflammation without affecting your mental abilities in the ways THC does.

Will CBD oil give you a high? Not without ample amounts of THC present. THC is marijuana's most famous ingredient, and when its psychoactive compounds are broken down by heat (either through smoking it or cooking it down into food), it provides that popular high. Unlike THC, CBD won't change your mental state or create feelings of intoxication.

Is CBD Oil Legal?

Understanding the legality of CBD oil in the U.S. is far from simple. Legislation regarding the substance differs at the state and federal levels, and marijuana laws are rarely straightforward, even in the states that have legalized it.

The legality of different cannabis products often comes down to whether the THC concentrations in

the original plant material classify it as hemp or marijuana. Currently, 34 states have laws that allow the cultivation of hemp for commercial, research, or pilot programs; 47 states (all except Idaho, Nebraska, and South Dakota) support the sale and use of hemp-derived CBD oil on at least a prescription basis. Eight states currently allow the recreational use and purchase of marijuana-derived CBD products, which include the mind-altering THC.

The process of purchasing the oil or acquiring a prescription varies by state. If CBD extracts are made from agricultural hemp and contain less than 0.3 percent THC, then the odds are good that they're legal to use and purchase where you live. But do your research carefully, as these rulings and their interpretations are regularly and rapidly changing.

Medicinal Benefits of CBD Oil

Considering the controversy over its legality, is CBD oil still worth pursuing? Researchers seem to think so. Decades of scientific studies show that CBD oil interacts with the body through a variety of biological processes that can reduce inflammation, boost relaxation, improve sleep, and more.

How to Use CBD Oil

Ready to give CBD oil a try? The way it should be used depends on the quality and concentration of your oil and what you're trying to treat. Some CBD products need to be mixed into food and drink, while others come as creams to be massaged into your skin. Still other CBD products come in capsules to be taken as a daily supplement. Below are some of the most popular forms this potent oil can take.

Capsules: CBD capsules are a simple way to incorporate CBD into your diet. Most pills can be taken daily, and offer 25 mg or less of CBD.

Concentrates: Designed to deliver a dose up to 10 times stronger than other CBD products, concentrates are typically taken via a dropper bottle in small amounts under your tongue.

Crystals: Isolated pure CBD crystals provide a versatile option for adding the compound to recipes or dissolving it into drinks. The crystallization process removes fats and lipids, leaving only the cannabinoids.

Sprays: At about 1 to 3 mg of CBD per serving, CBD sprays are typically the least concentrated form of the compound commercially available, making them an easy, flexible option, especially for new CBD users. You can spray servings directly into your mouth as needed.

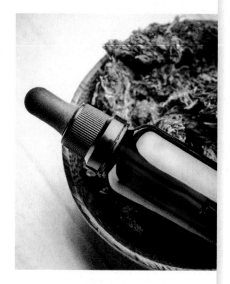

Tinctures: These strong CBD concentrations are meant to be taken just a few drops at a time. The longer you let the tincture sit under your tongue before swallowing, the stronger the benefits. It's also possible to add a dropperful of CBD tincture to hot water for an instant tea.

Topicals: Lotions, salves, serums, and balms can all contain CBD oil to improve their effectiveness for treating chronic pain, acne, and other health symptoms.

Before you turn to CBD oil for every ailment, keep in mind that few long-term studies have been conducted on its safety, and the compound hasn't yet been thoroughly tested on children. Consequently, the FDA hasn't approved CBD for any medical treatment at this time.

For this reason, talk with your doctor or dermatologist before beginning to experiment with CBD products. A health-care professional can also direct you to reputable brands and help you understand what dosage is best for your situation.

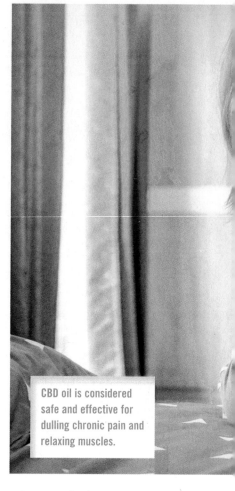

CBD oil is considered safe and effective for dulling chronic pain and relaxing muscles.

Some of the most prominent benefits of CBD oil include:

Natural pain relief: Pain relief is the most common use of medical marijuana in the U.S. Though CBD oil won't make much of a difference in severe pain such as a broken bone it's considered safe and effective for dulling chronic pain and relaxing muscles. Many people use it as a replacement for nonsteroidal anti-inflammatory drugs, including Advil and Aleve, to reduce the risk of compromising their kidneys.

Because of CBD's ability to ease pain from multiple sclerosis, nerve damage, and spinal cord injuries, many people prefer it to highly sedating and occasionally addictive opiates.

Epilepsy treatment: Thanks to its anti-seizure properties and low risk of side effects, CBD oil is considered a promising treatment option for epilepsy, especially in children. However, studies claiming this effect have been small,

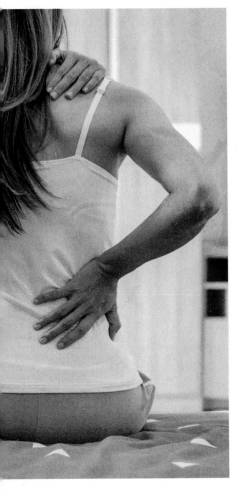

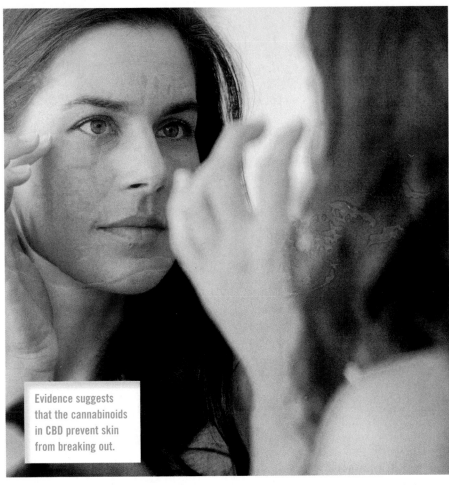

Evidence suggests that the cannabinoids in CBD prevent skin from breaking out.

randomized, and anecdotal, and further research is needed.

Neuroprotective properties: Because of the way CBD oil impacts neural receptors, evidence shows that it can benefit those with neurodegenerative disorders such as Alzheimer's disease, Parkinson's disease, and strokes. The oil seems especially helpful for preventing early-stage Alzheimer's patients from losing their ability to recognize faces. Further evidence shows CBD oil may also be useful in treating mental health disorders such as schizophrenia.

Acne prevention and solution: Because inflammation triggers acne, there's evidence that the cannabinoids in CBD prevent your skin from breaking out. Research shows that CBD can slow down production in the sebaceous glands to stop the skin from overproducing oil.

Reduction in withdrawal symptoms: Early evidence reveals that CBD oil

might help people quit smoking. One study of cigarette smokers who wished to quit showed that the participants who used an inhaler with CBD compounds experienced less-severe cravings for nicotine and smoked fewer cigarettes overall than those in the placebo group. A similar study found that the oil might be effective against opioid abuse withdrawal symptoms.

Natural cancer fighter: Research indicates that CBD might work as an anti-cancer agent by moderating inflammation, blocking cancer cells from spreading throughout the body, and causing them to die quickly. The National Cancer Institute states that CBD oil might be useful for suppressing cancer symptoms as well as the side effects from treatments.

Prevention of anxiety disorders: Research shows that CBD oil might lead to calming effects for people with post-traumatic stress disorder, general anxiety,

panic disorders, social anxiety disorder, and obsessive-compulsive disorder. According to initial reports, the oil can reduce symptoms of anxiety with fewer side effects than conventional medications because it naturally increases the brain's levels of serotonin.

Reduced risk of Type 1 diabetes: Type 1 diabetes is caused by the immune system attacking cells in the pancreas, which leads to chronic inflammation. Research shows that CBD might ease this inflammation and better control the body's response to the condition, which would keep those afflicted in better health. ✿

Lydia Noyes is a full-time freelance writer and former homesteader in central Appalachia. Today, she's working with her husband to start a small farm in southwest Michigan. You can find her online at FirstRootsFarm.com.

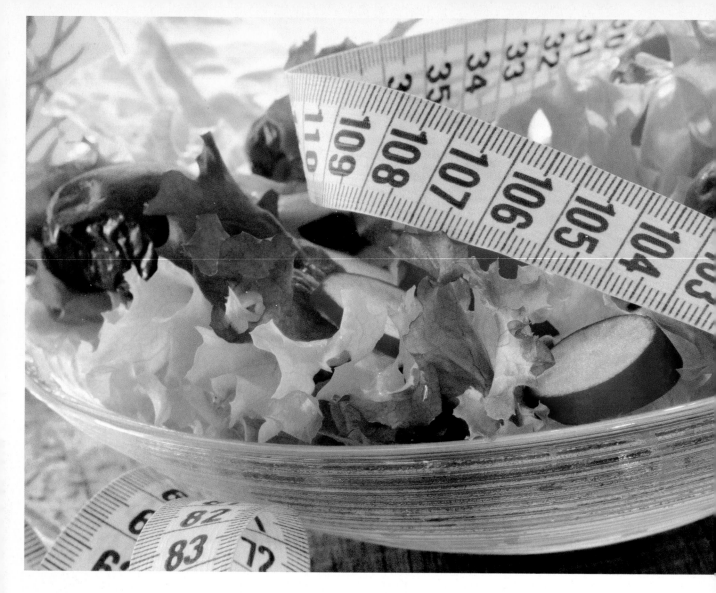

Live Leaner and Longer

Learn which herbs can boost metabolism, burn fat, and help you feel full.

By Linda B. White, M.D.

Forget the Fountain of Youth. While many red-blooded Americans would like to look forever young, the majority would rather fit into a pair of size 6 jeans. About 70 percent of American adults are overweight, and 40 percent are obese. "Globesity" has become an epidemic worldwide—even among children.

As it turns out, body weight does influence longevity. Ponce de Leon, the Spanish explorer who slogged around swampy Florida seeking the fabled Fountain, would have been fascinated by recent research from *The New England Journal of Medicine* showing that being even moderately overweight shortens life expectancy. Excess body fat also raises the risk of a host of maladies, including heart disease, atherosclerosis, high blood pressure, diabetes, osteoarthritis, depression, and some cancers.

Most of us know the risks. So why do our girths keep expanding? Experts blame several factors: the abundance of high-calorie (and not necessarily nutritious) food; super-sized portions; too much time sitting in front of computers and television screens; too little time moving our bodies; and suburban sprawl, which fosters a reliance on automobiles.

It all comes down to energy balance: the ratio of calories consumed versus calories burned. The solution? Eat less and exercise more—a simple plan many find difficult to impossible to follow. The keys to success lie in identifying your personal tar pits and making those small-but-powerful lifestyle changes you can stick with.

Look Deeper

To lose weight and keep it off, Brigitte Mars, a Boulder, Colorado-based herbalist and author of several books, including *Rawsome!* and *The Desktop Guide to Herbal Medicine*, says you must first examine and resolve the reasons you overeat. She asks her clients such questions as, "What was going on in your life when your weight became excessive?" or "Are you trying to armor or protect yourself from something?" She might also ask, "Are you using your weight as a way to bow out of social events and avoid intimate relationships?"

But reasons for overeating also can be more mundane, says Carrie Schroeder McConnell, a registered dietician who teaches nutrition at Metropolitan State College of Denver and has worked in an obesity clinic at the Children's Hospital in Denver. "We eat because someone else paid for it, because it tastes good, because we're encouraged by loved ones to eat, because we don't want to be rude, because we worry that if we don't eat that ice cream, someone else will," she says.

Likening excess body baggage to unnecessary personal possessions, Mars urges her clients literally to clean house. "Lighten your load by letting go of stuff you don't need," she says. "What you do on the outside sets the tone for what you're doing on the inside."

While you're cleaning your internal house, get rid of guilt. If you overindulge at a party, remain positive (but not delusional). Resolve to go for a longer hike the next day — then follow through and do it. Life is full of minor setbacks. Focus on long-term, slow, steady evolution. Documenting your progress will help you stay positive.

Get a Move On

Caloric restriction represents only half of the weight-loss equation. Successful weight loss requires exercise — the importance of this cannot be overstated. Whereas dieting can lower your metabolic rate (the rate at which your body burns calories), vigorous exercise increases it — for up to 12 hours afterward. Over time, physical exertion increases muscle tissue, which burns more calories than fat.

If you're new to exercise, build up gradually. Several short bursts of moderate exercise over the day add up. Pass up that great parking place for a more distant one. Take the stairs rather than the elevator. Take up gardening, tap dancing, or another activity you enjoy. The more you like it, the more you'll want to continue. McConnell recommends at least 30 to 60 minutes on most days of the week, noting that a survey by the National Weight Control Registry found that people who exercised 90 minutes a day were most likely to keep lost weight off. But don't be discouraged by the high number — you don't have to spend the whole time on a treadmill. Remember, all the forms of exercise you do throughout the day can add up to your 90 minutes.

My daughter, who worked in a bicycle store this summer, told me of a plump customer who exchanged her car for a new bike. She cycled everywhere — to work, to the store, and just for fun. A few months later, she had lost 60 pounds!

What About Herbs?

In 2001, Americans spent an estimated $2 billion on weight-loss supplements. According to Robert Saper, assistant professor and director of integrative medicine at Boston University Medical Center, "Only about half the ingredients in weight-loss supplements have undergone studies in humans, and none of these supplements has a robust amount of evidence demonstrating efficacy and safety." For that reason, he does not recommend them to his patients.

Max Pittler and Edzard Ernst, two researchers from England's Universities of Exeter and Plymouth, reviewed weight-loss supplements and concluded that their analyses, while "encouraging in some cases, provided little convincing evidence that any specific dietary supplement is effective in reducing body weight." Further, supplements that do appear to be effective can carry the risk of serious side effects.

Eric Yarnell, a Seattle-area naturopathic physician and

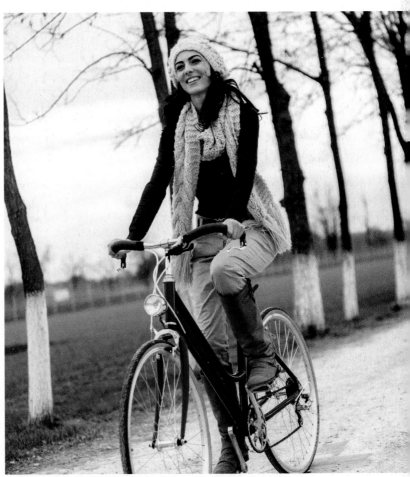

Whereas dieting can lower your metabolic rate, vigorous exercise increases it. Even just riding your bike in lieu of your car may help you shed pounds.

Best Tips for Long-Term Success

SET REASONABLE GOALS. If you vow to shed 5 pounds in one week, you will miss the mark or quickly regain the weight. Only unhealthful maneuvers (starvation, taking diuretics, purging) yield rapid weight loss. Losing weight and staying healthy will take time.

DON'T DEPRIVE YOURSELF. Eating fewer calories doesn't mean going hungry. Healthy foods are delicious and satisfying, says herbalist Brigitte Mars. "If you're satisfied, you don't overeat." Cold-turkeying your favorite, high-calorie foods may intensify cravings. If dinner isn't complete without dessert, satisfy that sweet tooth with a bite—a morsel of chocolate (rather than the whole bar) or a spoonful of ice cream (not the whole pint). People often are surprised to find they enjoy the first bite most, anyway.

STEER CLEAR OF EXTREME DIETS. From a weight-loss standpoint, it doesn't matter if you eat only bacon or grapefruit—as long as you limit your daily calorie intake. Your body stores extra calories as fat and doesn't care if they come from protein, carbohydrates, or fat. A 2005 study published in the *Journal of the American Medical Association* compared four diets: Atkins (low carbohydrate), Zone (balanced protein, carbs, and fats), Weight Watchers (caloric restriction), and Ornish (low-fat). At the end of the year, dieters in all groups lost an average of 6 pounds. Individual success was determined not by the type of diet, but adherence to the regime.

CHOOSE YOUR CARBOHYDRATES WISELY. "All carbohydrates provide four calories per gram," says dietician Carrie McConnell. "Regardless of whether your calories come from Gummy Bears or beans, you'll lose weight if you take in less than you expend." The difference is, the beans are more nutritious and high in fiber, which slows passage through the digestive tract and keeps you feeling full. Good carbs come from whole grains, fruits, and vegetables. And there is evidence that a plant-based diet improves weight loss. In a 2005 study published in *The American Medical Journal*, 64 overweight, postmenopausal women embarked on a low-fat, vegan diet. Their results? The women lost an average of nearly 13 pounds in 14 weeks — without being advised to limit calories.

DON'T FEAR GOOD FATS. Fats help you feel satisfied and full. "Bad" fats are solid at room temperature: especially trans, or hydrogenated, fats (found in many processed foods). "Good" fats are liquid at room temperature and include monounsaturated (olive oil) and polyunsaturated fats (most other vegetable oils and fish oils). Read labels. Be leery of products advertised as low-fat; they're often loaded with refined carbohydrates such as sugar and high-fructose corn syrup.

EAT SLOWLY AND WITH ATTENTION. If you munch while working or watching TV, you may not even notice how many chips you ate until your hand hits the bottom of the bag. The brain lags 20 minutes behind the stomach in registering fullness. So savor every bite—pause and appreciate smells, textures, and flavors. "Pay attention to those internal signals," McConnell says, "and stop when you're full."

DON'T SKIP MEALS. If you do, you'll be so famished the next time you sit at the dinner table you'll bolt your food and have trouble pushing away. "Healthy choices and portion control become extremely hard to practice when you're starving," McConnell says. Eat a good breakfast and make lunch your main meal. "We need more fuel in the daytime. In the evening, we usually eat dinner, then watch TV or read. Most of us just aren't active at night."

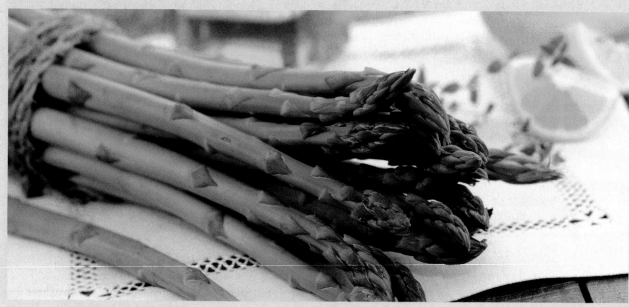

PLAN AHEAD. On Sunday, McConnell plans meals and shops for groceries for the entire week. "Healthy eating is more likely if it's convenient," she says. "Having good food on hand keeps you from snacking on junk food." McConnell keeps prepackaged yogurt shakes and fruit on hand for rushed mornings. To get through her busy day, she packs lunch and snackable vegetables such as baby carrots, sugar snap peas, and grape tomatoes.

DON'T OBSESS ON DIETING. When I was a medical student, I was fascinated with eating disorders—an interest that no doubt stemmed from my years in mirrored ballet studios. My senior thesis examined factors that helped teens lose weight. The "successful losers" had developed an interest that took their minds off food. One joined a theater group. Another started dating. A third teen took up in-line skating.

SPEND LESS TIME STARING AT ELECTRONIC SCREENS. Several studies have shown a correlation between hours spent in front of the TV and weight gain. Go outside. Or exercise while you watch. If you sit at a computer terminal all day, take frequent breaks to get up and move around.

SLEEP ON IT AND STRESS LESS. Both sleep deprivation and stress overload contribute to weight gain. One study found that women who slept less than seven hours a night were more likely to gain weight. Conversely, getting sufficient sleep lowers the risk. Sleep deprivation decreases the hormone leptin and increases ghrelin, leading to slowed metabolism and a heightened appetite. Furthermore, insufficient sleep stresses the body. Any kind of stress elevates the hormone cortisol, which breaks down muscle protein, deposits fat in the belly, and stimulates appetite. Plus, who feels like exercising when tired and stressed out? It all works together: Managing stress ensures good sleep, and exercise and proper nutrition relieve stress.

DRINK UNSWEETENED BEVERAGES. A can of soda a day (which contains 10 teaspoons of sugar) can tip the scales 15 pounds by year's end, according to a 2004 study published in *JAMA*. Other beverages to minimize include juice and beverages sweetened with high-fructose corn syrup or sugar. Instead, drink water and unsweetened tea or coffee. A bit of low-fat milk or soy milk in your coffee is fine and will provide calcium. A tall glass of water before a meal will make your stomach feel full sooner and improve bowel function.

REWARD YOURSELF. Losing unwanted pounds is reward in itself. Bask in those compliments you'll soon hear. Give yourself motivating treats: a membership at an athletic club at the start; a massage after 5 pounds; a new dress when you're down 10 pounds; a spa weekend at 15 pounds. Try not to think of rich food as a reward.

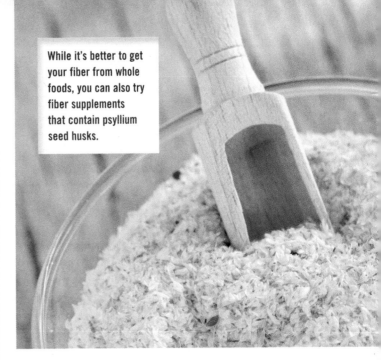

While it's better to get your fiber from whole foods, you can also try fiber supplements that contain psyllium seed husks.

assistant professor at Bastyr University, recommends herbal supplements only to his patients who already are making serious attempts to exercise and improve their diets. "Weight-loss supplements are only crutches, not magical solutions," he says. "If one doesn't reduce one's intake of calories and increase one's use of calories, then no herb in the world is ultimately going to work for more than a short period of time and may cause a lot of problems in the meantime."

Some herbs add fiber, rev up your metabolism, burn fat, and suppress appetite (see the following examples). "Most of these herbs are safe used in reasonable doses for most basically healthy people," Yarnell says. "They are only a problem when people start overdosing to be super athletes or if they believe they can melt off the fat with a pill."

Herbs that Help You Feel Full

Plants high in soluble fiber absorb water, making you feel full. Provided you stop eating when you feel full, you will theoretically consume fewer calories. Other benefits of soluble fiber in the diet include improved bowel regularity and reduced blood levels of cholesterol and glucose (sugar). These latter two actions reduce the risk of atherosclerosis and diabetes, respectively. Common foods rich in soluble fiber include legumes, oats, barley, and fruits such as apples and citrus.

While experts such as Yarnell and Mars say it's better to get your fiber from whole foods, you will find plenty of fiber supplements on the market. These products typically contain glucomannan, which is derived from konjac root (*Amorphophallus konjac*), guar gum, a common thickening agent derived from the seeds of the Indian cluster bean (*Cyamopsis tetragonoloba*) or psyllium seed husks (*Plantago* spp.).

These fiber supplements generally are safe, although effectiveness varies. Four small trials suggest glucomannan may help, whereas the other two fiber forms haven't proven successful. Saper speculates that glucomannon may have specific characteristics that differ from soluble fiber in common

Avoid These Herbal Supplements

Don't take herbal laxatives such as senna *(Senna alexandrina)* or cascara sagrada *(Rhamnus purshiana)* to lose weight; what's lost are water and electrolytes, not fat. Dandelion increases water loss from the kidneys; unlike pharmaceutical diuretics, dandelion doesn't deplete the body of potassium—but, once again, the goal is to lose unsightly fat, not life-promoting water.

Important note: Even if you think you're healthy, discontinue a weight-loss product if you notice insomnia, jitteriness, racing heart rate, or palpitations. And please don't combine such products with decongestant-containing cold preparations or stimulants to treat attention deficit disorder. If you're pregnant or nursing, avoid all strong herbs and drugs.

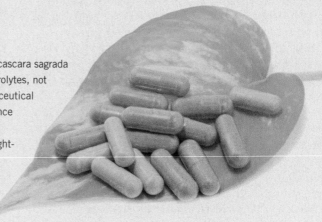

foods. Study doses of glucomannan average 3 to 4 grams a day, divided into three doses and taken with a tall glass of water an hour before each meal. To avoid bothersome symptoms such as flatulence, bloating, indigestion, and nausea, start with a low dose and gradually increase.

Calorie-Burning Herbs?

Thermogenesis means generating heat. The body heats itself by expending energy and burning calories. Thermogenic substances favor the conversion of food into heat rather than fat. Examples of such substances include plants that contain stimulant alkaloids such as caffeine, ephedrine, and synephrine. The latter two chemicals also may reduce food intake. Coffee, black and green tea, guarana *(Paullinia cupana)*, and yerba maté *(Ilex paraguariensis)* all contain caffeine. Bitter orange *(Citrus limetta)* contains synephrine and octopamine. Cinnamon, ginger, garlic, and cayenne improve circulation and safely warm the body, Mars says.

While research suggests that these alkaloids can improve weight loss, they also stimulate the cardiovascular, respiratory, and nervous systems. In excess, they can cause jitteriness, insomnia, upset stomach, palpitations, rapid heart rate, and elevated blood pressure. (For example, ephedra—an herb that was once sold as a weight-loss supplement—can trigger heart attacks, seizures, and strokes. Such adverse events caused the FDA to remove ephedra from the market in 2004.)

Lately, bitter orange has become a popular weight-loss supplement, although there is not enough scientific evidence to support this use. Also known as Seville orange, the fruit of this spiny evergreen tree is used to make marmalade, the liqueurs Triple Sec and curaçao, and orange flower water. It yields neroli and bergamot, essential oils prized by aromatherapists and perfumers. Traditional Chinese Medicine practitioners call it *zhi shi* and use it for gastrointestinal ailments.

Bitter orange contains synephrine and optopamine, weaker chemical cousins to ephedrine and adrenaline (also known as epinephrine) and norepinephrine, which are manufactured by the body. A pharmaceutical derivation of synephrine, phenylephrine (Neosynephrine) is used to treat nasal congestion and low blood pressure.

A recent review of the research on bitter orange extracts for weight loss, published in *Obesity Reviews* in 2006, labeled the preliminary evidence "promising" and called for further investigation. Of the four studies demonstrating significant weight loss, all were of short duration (two to six weeks) and used small numbers of volunteers (nine to 30 people). None tested bitter orange alone. Rather, bitter orange extract was variously combined with caffeine, guarana, ginkgo, and St. John's wort. Effects of these products on heart rate and blood pressure were mixed.

The safety of bitter orange is not clear-cut. The herb's active ingredients, synephrine and octopamine, are not well-absorbed from the digestive tract and are weaker than ephedrine. Studies have used synephrine alkaloids in daily doses as low as 5 mg (in combination with caffeine and ephedrine) and up to 120 mg (used alone). Christine Haller, an assistant professor in the department of medicine at the University of California, San Francisco, notes, "It is unusual to find a commercial product that only contains bitter orange." Bitter orange also contains chemicals that may speed up heart rate and raise blood pressure, so talk to your health-care provider before deciding to take this herb as a dietary supplement. Pregnant women or nursing mothers should avoid bitter orange due to lack of safety evidence.

Fat-Burning Herbs

In addition to being thermogenic, green tea stimulates fat breakdown. Tea contains caffeine and flavonoids called catechins, which act synergistically. To illustrate this interaction, researchers gave 10 healthy men either green tea extract

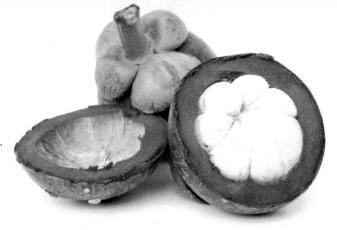

(50 mg caffeine and 90 mg epigallocatechin gallate), caffeine alone (50 mg), or a placebo pill. Only the green tea extract significantly increased 24-hour energy expenditure (a measurement of calories burned)—without raising heart rate.

However, a 2005 study published in the *British Journal of Nutrition* found that adding green tea extract (providing 1,125 mg tea catechins and 225 mg caffeine a day) to a low-calorie diet didn't augment long-term weight loss in a group of women, though it did counteract the dip in energy expenditure that comes with restricting calories. At this point, there isn't enough research to judge green tea's weight-loss power.

A plant-derived supplement called hydroxycitric acid (HCA) alters fat metabolism by both inhibiting fat production and promoting its breakdown; it also reduces appetite. HCA is extracted from the rind of a pumpkin-shaped fruit native to Indonesia known as garcinia (*Garcinia cambogia*), also called brindleberry or Malabar tamarind. In a review of herb safety, Pittler and Ernst found garcinia was one of the few supplements—with preliminary scientific support—that appeared to be safe. While one study failed to find benefit, three studies demonstrated weight loss, although one of them didn't find that HCA curbed appetite. Another study failed to confirm that HCA significantly altered energy expenditure or fat metabolism.

Two of the positive trials used a product said to be more bioavailable called HCA-SX, providing 2,800 to 4,667 mg a day of HCA, divided into three doses and taken 30 minutes before mealtime. This product is marketed as Super CitriMax, with a manufacturer's recommended dosage of 900 mg, 30 to

Garcinia may be a safe supplement to aid in weight loss.

60 minutes before breakfast, lunch, and dinner. This supplement is not a ground herb but rather a chemical extracted from a plant.

Long-term safety for garcinia is still unknown, so be sure to talk with your health-care provider before deciding to take it.

Herbal Appetite Suppressants

Making a big media splash is hoodia (Hoodia gordonii), which has been featured on *Today* and *60 Minutes,* and in *O, The Oprah Magazine.* This rare succulent from the Kalahari Desert of South Africa has helped the Bushmen endure lean times and contains steroidal glycosides that trick the brain into thinking the stomach's full, thereby suppressing appetite—but without stimulating the cardiovascular and nervous systems. A substance isolated from hoodia called P57 has shown to suppress appetite and stimulate weight loss in laboratory animals.

In an unpublished study funded by the product's manufacturer, Phytopharm, 19 obese adults took either a placebo or a hoodia extract without changing diet or activity levels. After 15 days, the hoodia group had reduced their food intake by 1,000 calories a day—a big drop when you consider the average American needs around 2,200 calories per day.

Not all products that claim to contain hoodia really do, so make sure you have the real deal. Until the plant is mass cultivated, hoodia pills and liquid extracts will remain rare and expensive. More scientific evidence is still needed before supporting this herb's effectiveness and safety, so be sure to talk with your health-care provider before deciding to take hoodia.

Reaching Your Own Bottom Line

What does this all mean for the average person trying to shed flab? Eat fewer calories and make sure those calories are nutrient- and fiber-rich. Exercise every day. And hold off on weight-loss supplements until there's enough research to prove they're both effective and safe. As Ponce de Leon learned long ago, there is no magic potion. 🌳

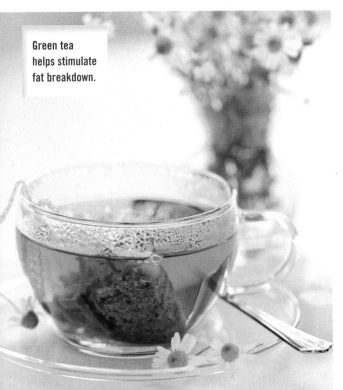

Green tea helps stimulate fat breakdown.

Linda B. White, M.D., is the author of *500 Time-Tested Home Remedies* (available at MotherEarthNews.com/Store). A plant-based diet and daily rambles with her dog help keep her lean.

Graceful

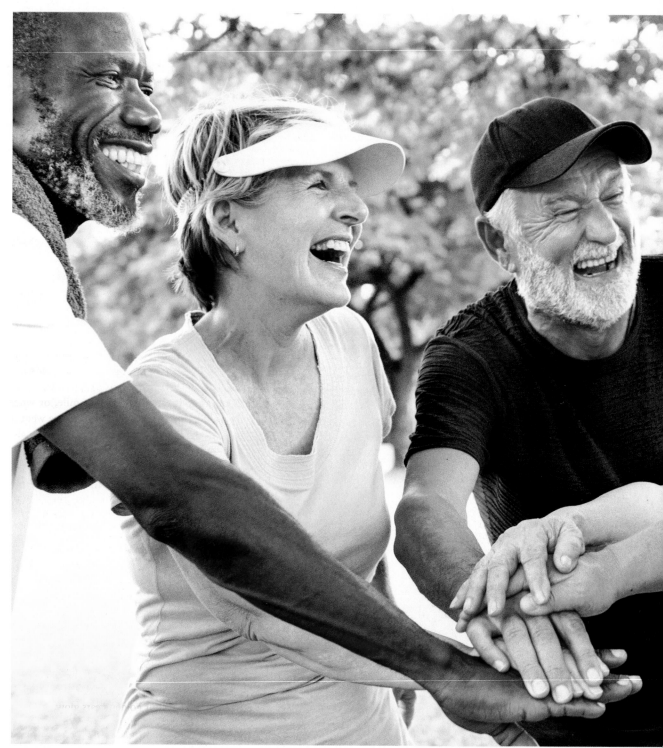

Aging

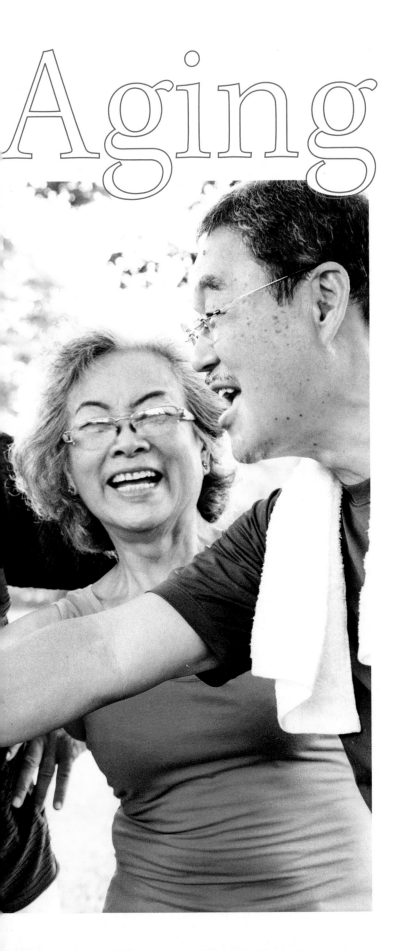

Although getting older makes us wiser, it also comes with a few common complaints — aches, pains, drier skin, and increased forgetfulness, to name a few. Make your golden years glow brighter with these tips, habits, and recipes that can help ward off the ailments of aging — at any age.

By *Mother Earth Living* editors

Most people complain about the symptoms of aging from time to time, whether it's when we notice an uptick in the time it takes us to run a mile, or when we walk into a room and forget why we went in there in the first place. But growing older is also wonderful. Every day, month, and year we're alive is another opportunity to create new memories with our friends and families; to improve our knitting, painting, pie-baking, or card-playing skills; to travel somewhere we've never been; or to watch our children or grandchildren or nieces and nephews grow. Yet the joys of these moments can be tempered by the ailments of growing older. Wrestling with your grandson is a little less fun when you have chronic shoulder pain. And a night out with our best friends is always more fun when we feel we look our best (and don't have to spend the whole night seeking the nearest bathroom!). The recommendations throughout this article are all backed up by research or experts in their field. We hope some of them will come in handy to make your golden years glow.

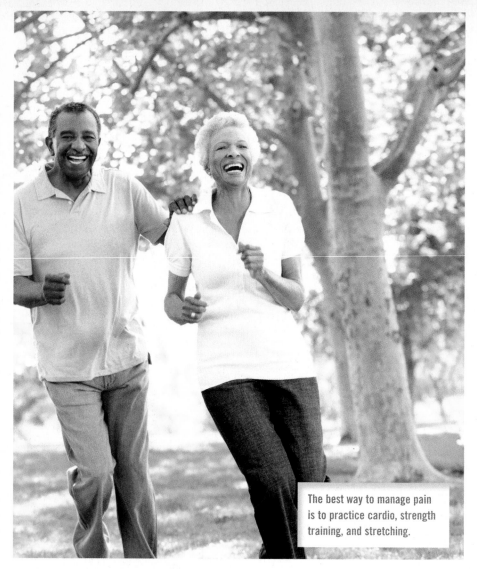

The best way to manage pain is to practice cardio, strength training, and stretching.

Aches & Pains

Aches and pains are a common complaint of aging, although chronic pain can afflict adults of all ages. Some of the most widely reported types of pain include joint and muscle pain. This can be caused by arthritis, but also simply because our ligaments, muscles, and tendons become less pliant as we age, leading to aching and soreness. One of the best ways to combat aching joints is to commit to building and maintaining flexibility. Stephanie Siegrist, a doctor and the author of *Know Your Bones: Making Sense of Arthritis Medicine*, suggests the best way to manage pain is to consider ideal conditioning as a three-legged stool, consisting of cardio (especially important to keep weight down, which will improve joint health); strength training (to maintain muscle density; stronger muscles also help keep ligaments and tendons aligned); and flexibility (which means daily stretching or yoga). She recommends older adults focus equal attention on all three—and never give flexibility short shrift. If back pain is a problem (lower back pain is the most commonly reported type of pain in the U.S.), focus on exercises that strengthen the core. That can include upright cardiovascular exercises such as jogging, as well as core-strengthening workouts such as Pilates and yoga. Consult with your health-care practitioner to determine whether any pain medication, supplement, or technique is appropriate for you—especially if you have any significant health issues.

Herbal remedies can also offer a natural way to manage aches and pains. Unlike over-the-counter and prescription medication, many natural herbal remedies are safe to take daily over the long term. For arthritis pain, famed herbalist James Duke recommends standardized extracts of boswellia, derived from the same tree that produces frankincense. Devil's claw, turmeric, and ginger are other highly anti-inflammatory herbs frequently used to treat arthritis pain. Look for high-quality supplements or teas at health-food stores and follow label dosing instructions, or consult a certified herbalist or naturopathic doctor who can develop an herbal program specifically for you. Taking omega-3 fatty acid supplements, as well as glucosamine and the naturally occurring methylsulfonylmethane (MSM), are also supported by research. Don't combine MSM with blood thinners.

Finally, massage, acupuncture, and water therapy (bathing or hot tubs) are all research-backed ways to help manage pain. Several types of massage are recommended to help manage pain, according to the Arthritis Foundation. Try combining regular professional massage with daily self-massage. Massage is also beneficial to aid in sleep, which is a problem for many arthritis sufferers. Massage can promote deep sleep, which is when the body is most able to recover. And although acupuncture is somewhat controversial, its most well-researched benefit is pain management. In a study of nearly 18,000 patients published in the *Archives of Internal Medicine*, researchers found acupuncture outperformed sham treatments and standard care in people suffering osteoarthritis, migraines, and chronic back, neck, and shoulder pain. When it comes to bathing, opt for 20 minutes in warm (92- to 100-degree) water, and do some gentle stretching while the water is loosening your muscles.

The Anatomy of Pain

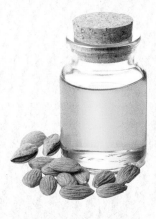

We all know what pain feels like, but few of us know the biology behind the "ouch" factor. Pain is a result of inflammation. When we are injured, the body responds with cyclooxygenase-2 (COX-2), a relatively recently discovered enzyme related to COX-1. While COX-1 enzymes are responsible for maintaining balance in the stomach and kidneys, COX-2 involves turning a stored fat called arachidonic acid into prostaglandins, which inflame injured areas and lead to pain.

Enter nonsteroidal anti-inflammatory drugs (NSAIDs) such as aspirin, ibuprofen, or naproxen, over-the-counter remedies that work by inhibiting COX-1 and COX-2 enzymes. Although NSAIDs are the most popular pain-relief medications, long-term use can result in gastrointestinal upset, peptic ulcers, and intestinal bleeding, and may even contribute to colon, kidney, or liver damage. In fact, a report in *The American Journal of Medicine* revealed that more than 107,000 people are hospitalized each year due to complications from NSAID use.

In an effort to soothe pain without leaving users vulnerable to these side effects, researchers created a new generation of COX-2 inhibitors. Sold under the names Celebrex and Vioxx, these drugs also relieve pain and inflammation, but because they only target the COX-2 enzyme, they carry fewer gastrointestinal risks than traditional NSAIDs. Better yet, studies found that Celebrex was just as effective at stopping pain as narcotics without the risk of addiction, and Vioxx could conquer the toughest menstrual cramps. But while these drugs were being hailed as the new "safe" aspirin, reports began to surface of side effects, including diarrhea, headaches, respiratory infections, dizziness, and skin rashes. Researchers from the University of California at Irvine found these new pain relievers could worsen colitis and interfere with the healing of gastric ulcers. Of greater concern, the FDA received reports of 10 deaths within months of the release of Celebrex. Vioxx was removed from the market in 2004. Celebrex remains a popular arthritis drug.

A widely reported, large-scale study published in the *New England Journal of Medicine* in 2016 compared celecoxib (Celebrex), ibuprofen, and naproxen, and found Celebrex was safer than both ibuprofen and naproxen when used long-term—although some experts cite study weaknesses, including a low inclusion of patients with heart disease (the most worrisome) and a high patient drop-out rate, making data interpretation difficult. Of the study, Dr. Elliott Antman, a professor of medicine at Harvard Medical School and a past president of the American Heart Association, said he would continue to advise that any of the drugs in the study be taken only by the lowest-risk patients and in the lowest dose possible for the shortest time possible. Another doctor, Michael Joseph Blaha, director of clinical research for the Johns Hopkins Ciccarone Center for the Prevention of Heart Disease, says: "I would not feel comfortable saying it is perfectly safe to take celecoxib. But if you need to take a daily pill it might be safer to take this one than (ibuprofen or naproxen)."

Kim Erickson; updated by the editors

Arthritis-Relief Rub
This simple recipe may help soothe pain and inflammation in the joints.

Ingredients
- 2 tablespoons carrier oil such as almond or jojoba
- 10 drops lavender essential oil
- 10 drops rosemary essential oil

Directions: Combine ingredients and rub gently onto painful areas twice daily. Do not use on large areas of the body.

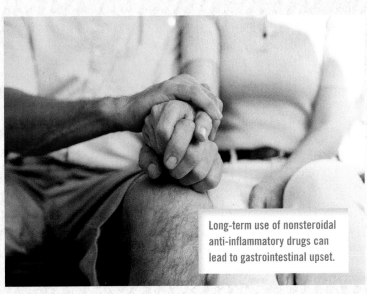

Long-term use of nonsteroidal anti-inflammatory drugs can lead to gastrointestinal upset.

Magic Erasers

- If you're looking to eliminate age spots, try these natural remedies, found as close as your pantry or refrigerator.

- The high acid content in apple cider vinegar makes it an excellent skin exfoliant. Dab some on your age spots before bedtime. If the solution stings, leave the vinegar on for 30 minutes and then wash it off.

- Apply freshly squeezed lemon juice to age spots twice daily for a few months. The citric acid in lemons provides a natural bleaching agent that can diminish the appearance of the spots.

- Raw fruit such as papaya pulp and pineapple contain enzymes that can accelerate skin exfoliation when used over time. Dab onto skin with a cotton ball.

- Yogurt contains lactic acid, which can lighten and exfoliate skin. Apply a thin layer of yogurt to age spots and let sit for 20 to 30 minutes.

Susan Melgren

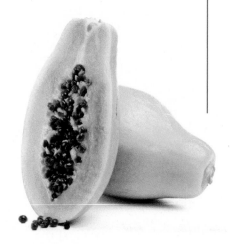

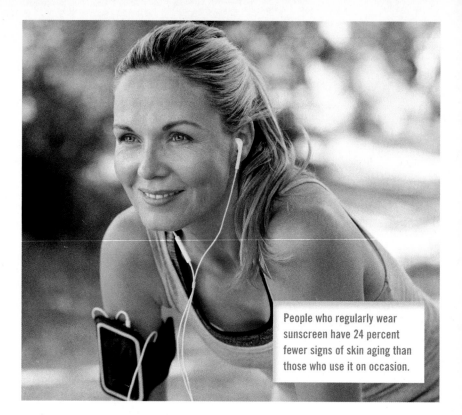

People who regularly wear sunscreen have 24 percent fewer signs of skin aging than those who use it on occasion.

Skin & Hair

As we age, our skin and hair can suffer from increased dryness and damage. Consider these tips to maintain your hair and skin's youthful appearance.

For skin, an anti-aging regimen should consist of these broad approaches.

Protect: Sunscreen is one of the most important ways we can maintain younger-looking skin. People who regularly apply sunscreen have 24 percent fewer signs of skin aging than those who only use sunscreen on occasion, according to a study published in the *Annals of Internal Medicine*. But all sunscreen is not necessarily equal: Avoid sunscreens made with vitamin A; estrogen-mimicking oxybenzone; and SPFs higher than 50, which research indicates may not actually provide additional protection. Opt for a mineral-based natural sunscreen that lists micronized zinc and titanium dioxide as its active ingredients, at SPF 30. Learn more about the best brands at EWG.org/Sunscreen.

Exfoliate: Because it sloughs away dead skin cells and unclogs oil and dirt from pores, exfoliation is particularly important for aging skin. As our skin ages, the natural exfoliation process slows and dry cells linger longer on the surface. Gently exfoliate mature skin once or twice a week with natural particles such as sugar, nuts, or seeds. (Salt is typically too abrasive for facial skin.) Avoid products with plastic microbeads. These scrubber fragments move through drains and into the ocean, where they have become a concern to marine life.

Moisturize: As we age, our top layer of skin can dry and form microscopic cracks that make it more irritable and prone to inflammation. Regular application of moisturizers with natural emollients and ingredients can help: A popular active ingredient in anti-aging moisturizers, coenzyme Q10 may improve skin's texture and elasticity, boost collagen production, and ward off free radicals. Indian frankincense extract, also known as *Boswellia serrata*, has anti-inflammatory properties and may help reduce wrinkles. Vitamin B3, often called niacin or niacinamide on product labels, boosts hydration and reduces redness.

Healthy Hair

Many of us notice changes in our hair as we age. Hair can become thinner in men and women, and it can also become more dry and brittle. Try these natural tips to maintain hair thickness and health.

• Saw palmetto is a well-studied herb used extensively for enlarged prostate in men. Saw palmetto is known to block the formation of the hormone DHT that is linked to male pattern baldness. It's generally taken in extract or tincture form.

• Licorice also contains a compound that prevents the conversion of testosterone to DHT. Medicinal plant expert James Duke recommends balding men add this herb to their favorite shampoo.

• Rosemary is an age-old remedy for healthy hair. Rosemary essential oil is often used, diluted in oil, for nightly scalp massages to increase circulation and stimulate hair growth. An infusion of rosemary can also be used as a rinse after shampooing.

• Horsetail has a high silica content and is included in many hair formulas. It's also sometimes used in the treatment of enlarged prostate. **Note:** Horsetail should not be combined with regular alcohol consumption.

• Nettle is rich in minerals that promote good circulation to the scalp and is used in Europe to help prevent balding. It can be taken as a tea or tincture.

• Arginine is an essential amino acid important to hair growth. The body uses it to form nitric oxide, a substance that stimulates hair growth. Arginine also may stimulate growth hormones that help prevent hair loss. It occurs naturally in meat, nuts, eggs, dairy products, wheat germ, and—in its highest quantities—sunflower seeds. It's available in tablet form, but don't take this in high doses or for prolonged periods. It's best to consult a physician before taking this amino acid in supplemental doses.

• L-cysteine is a common ingredient in hair formulas on the market. It's an amino acid found in many body proteins and is essential for proper hair growth. L-cysteine can build up in the body to toxic levels so, as with any medication, work with a health practitioner and follow dosage instructions.

• B vitamins, specifically biotin and B6, are included in most of the expensive hair regrowth formulas available in stores. These vitamins are coenzymes involved in the metabolism of proteins, and a deficiency of biotin may cause hair loss. Taking a good multivitamin will ensure you're getting enough B vitamins. B6 may also inhibit the creation of DHT.

• Oil massages may help stimulate hair growth. Make sure to use an all-natural oil and never synthetic, petroleum-based oils; castor oil is often recommended for hair growth. Combine the oil with a few drops of essential oils for greater effect. For dry or damaged hair, mix the following oils in 2 tablespoons oil: 1 drop cedar, 3 drops clary sage, 1 drop geranium, 1 drop lavender, and 3 drops rosemary. Massage into your scalp and hair, leave on for one hour or longer, then shampoo. For hair loss, use 3 drops cedar, 2 drops clary sage, 2 drops lemon, and 3 drops rosemary.

DIY Anti-Aging Cream

This evening face and neck cream is rich in skin-conditioning oils. For soft, smooth skin, massage a small amount into your face and neck nightly.

Ingredients

• 2 tablespoons coconut oil
• 1 tablespoon olive oil
• 1 tablespoon grated cocoa butter
• 1 teaspoon vitamin E oil

Directions: Mix all ingredients in a small pan and heat gently on the stovetop until mixture warms and just begins to melt.

Remove from heat and stir until completely melted and mixed. Pour into a clean jar with a lid.

To use, massage a small amount into your neck and face at night before going to bed.

Janice Cox

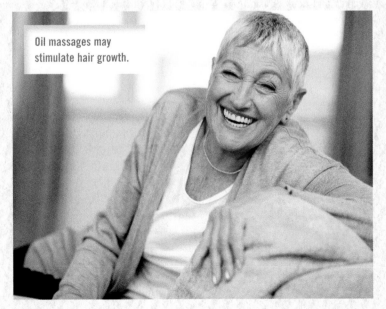

Oil massages may stimulate hair growth.

Bladder & Prostate Health

Bladder strength and urination can become issues as we age. The National Institute on Aging lists the causes of incontinence as weak or overactive bladder muscles; damage to nerves from diseases such as Parkinson's disease; blockage from an enlarged prostate in men; and diseases such as arthritis, which can make it difficult to reach the bathroom quickly.

Doing Kegel exercises is a great method of incontinence prevention. They can strengthen muscles and work best when practiced early in the onset of urinary issues. To do them, locate your pelvic muscles by stopping the flow of urine midstream. Empty your bladder, lie down, then squeeze and hold these muscles for a count of three; relax for a count of three. Do this 10 times; work up to three sets of 10 daily.

Lifestyle changes can also help improve bladder function. Excess weight can be a cause of bladder stress and can increase risk of incontinence, as can bladder irritants, including tobacco, caffeine, alcohol, black pepper, and other spices, according to famed physician Andrew Weil. Smoking is a particular risk—incontinence is twice as likely among smokers as it is among nonsmokers. Weil also recommends discussing bladder retraining programs with your physician. In these programs, you schedule a regular time to go to the bathroom (such as hourly), then gradually increase the interval between bathroom visits. Keeping a bladder diary may be a useful short-term tool to help reveal triggers and patterns.

> ## "Regular aerobic exercise appears to boost the size of the brain's hippocampus."

If these interventions don't work, you may wish to seek more complex treatments. In biofeedback therapy, sensors are used to make patients aware of signals from the body, helping regain muscle control. To find therapists, contact the Biofeedback Certification International Alliance at BCIA.org. Prescription options also exist for incontinence. They are frequently effective and can cause side effects such as dry mouth, constipation, blurred vision, and eye problems. They're not recommended for people with glaucoma, urinary retention, or gastrointestinal diseases. Your doctor may also suggest surgery.

Prostate Health

For older men, urinary issues are often tied to an enlarged prostate. After age 25, men's prostates begin to grow, due to benign prostatic hyperplasia (BPH). BPH causes no symptoms in 50 to 60 percent of men. But BPH can lead to symptoms, including hesitated, interrupted, or weak urine streams; urgency; leaking or dribbling urine; a sense of incomplete emptying; or more frequent urination at night. The Harvard Medical School recommends the following: Reduce stress by exercising regularly and practicing meditation; take the time to completely empty the bladder; talk with your doctor about prescription or over-the-counter medications that can contribute to the problem; and avoid drinking fluids at night, particularly caffeinated and alcoholic beverages. Finally, saw palmetto is an herb frequently recommended for prostate health. Although evidence is mixed on its effectiveness, several studies suggest it's effective for treating symptoms, according to the University of Maryland Medical Center. A few have found saw palmetto as effective as the prescription alternative, and others have suggested it may help shrink the prostate. Because many of these studies have been small and/or short, more research is needed. To try saw palmetto, find a high-quality supplement and follow label instructions.

Memory

Most people report age-related memory changes and an uptick in forgetfulness. Changes such as taking longer to learn new things, or forgetting where we set our keys are not a sign of serious problems. Some memory loss can be due to treatable issues such as medication side effects, vitamin B12 deficiency, or infections in the brain.

More severe types of memory problems include amnestic mild cognitive impairment (MCI). People suffering from amnestic MCI have more memory issues than normal but their symptoms aren't as severe as those with dementia or Alzheimer's disease, and they can carry out normal daily activities. People with amnestic MCI are more likely to develop Alzheimer's than those without, but not all amnestic MCI patients develop Alzheimer's. Dementia is a loss of memory, thinking, and reasoning skills that seriously disrupts daily life. Alzheimer's can cause dementia, as can other disorders. The National Institutes of Health lists the symptoms of dementia as: being unable to remember things; asking the same question or repeating the same story over and over; becoming lost in familiar places; being unable to follow directions; getting confused about time, people, and places; and neglecting personal safety, hygiene, and nutrition. Seek a health professional if you believe you or a loved one is suffering from a serious form of memory loss. 🌳

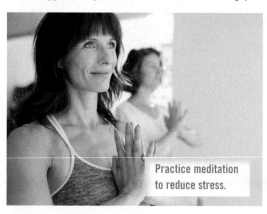

Practice meditation to reduce stress.

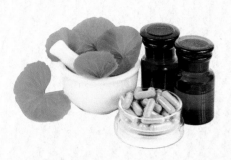

Herbs for Memory

Need a mental boost? The following are a few of the best time-tested herbs to help improve memory.

Ginkgo: Along with ginkgo's usefulness for memory loss, studies have confirmed its effectiveness for mental fatigue, senile dementia, and an inability to concentrate. Ginkgo improves blood supply to the brain, increases the brain's ability to use oxygen, and increases glucose uptake and energy production, thereby increasing aptitude and alertness. A commonly recommended dose is three capsules containing at least 40 mg of standardized extract daily—or follow the manufacturer's or your practitioner's recommendations. It often takes about two months to notice ginkgo's effects.

Gotu kola: This herb has a longstanding reputation as a memory herb. It's used in both Ayurvedic and Traditional Chinese Medicine, as well as by Western herbalists, for longevity and to improve mental function.

Rosemary: Rosemary contains more than a dozen antioxidants as well as several compounds that help prevent the breakdown of the neurotransmitter acetylcholine. Noted herbalist James Duke recommends using rosemary in shampoos and baths for its aromatherapeutic effects. You can make your own rosemary shampoo by adding a few drops of the pure essential oil to your shampoo bottle.

Remember This!

Try these research-backed ways to keep your memory sharp.

Engage in physical activity and exercise.

Several studies have associated physical activity with improved brain function. In one study at the University of British Columbia, researchers found that regular aerobic exercise appears to boost the size of the brain's hippocampus, responsible for verbal memory and learning.

Learn a new language.

People who speak more than two languages may lower their risk of developing memory problems, according to research from the Public Research Center for Health in Luxembourg.

Play games, read books, do crafts.

In a 2011 study published in *The Journal of Neuropsychiatry and Clinical Neurosciences*, scientists found leisure activities, including playing games, reading books, and crafting, were able to reduce chances of developing mild cognitive impairment by 30 to 50 percent.

Play an instrument.

In a 2011 study, people who spent at least 10 years playing an instrument scored highest on a comprehensive battery of neuropsychological tests, including nonverbal and visuospatial memory, naming objects, and taking in and adapting new information.

Limit alcohol use.

Although some studies suggest moderate alcohol consumption has health benefits, heavy or binge drinking over time can lead to memory loss and brain damage.

Play video games.

Yes, you read that right. In England, members of the BBC Horizon program recruited a group of elderly volunteers to learn to play a popular driving game, logging around 15 hours of game time over the course of five weeks. Their working memories and attention spans were tested before and after, and both scores increased by about 30 percent on average.

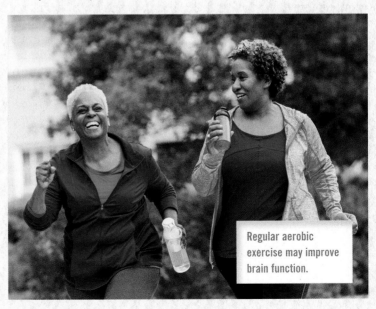

Regular aerobic exercise may improve brain function.

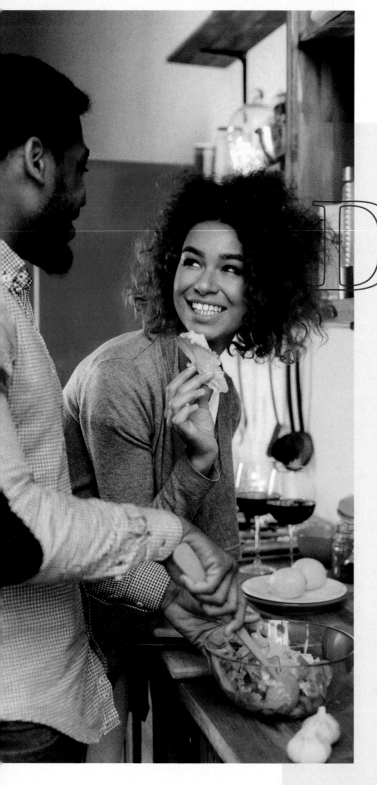

Readers, Digest

Use these simple, natural tips to keep the irritating symptoms of intestinal upset at bay.

By Linda B. White

Nausea, vomiting, heartburn, diarrhea, cramping, bloating, flatulence. We've all endured intestinal upset — sometimes at supremely inopportune moments. Digestive distress can manifest on airplanes, during business meetings, on bus trips in foreign lands, during a first date, while running a marathon, and even on stage.

Although some of us have more sensitive systems than others, we all have control over a number of factors that influence our digestive health. Try the following tips to keep your system running smoothly.

Eat Mainly Plants

Plant chemicals and nutrients promote overall health and protect against cancer, inflammation, and free radical damage. On the other hand, processed meat and red meat, especially meat cooked at high temperatures, is associated with an increased risk of colorectal cancer.

Plant-based diets also provide fiber, which, combined with plenty of fluids, prevents constipation. There are two types of fiber: insoluble and soluble. Insoluble fiber doesn't dissolve in water and passes through the intestinal tract unaltered. Sources include whole grains (whole wheat, brown rice, barley, farro, bulgur, and couscous), popcorn, lentils, dark green leafy vegetables, broccoli, cabbage, and celery.

Soluble fiber dissolves in water to form a gel, which slows digestion and enhances feelings of satiety. Bacteria that normally inhabit the intestinal tract ferment the gel, which promotes bowel health. Sources include oats, barley, beans, flax seeds, psyllium seed husks, nuts, carrots, apples, oranges, pears, strawberries, and blueberries.

According to one study, for people with irritable bowel system (IBS), soluble fiber appears to alleviate symptoms, while insoluble fiber may do the opposite. Consult your physician to consider whether reducing insoluble fiber may be helpful.

Rule Out Food Allergies and Intolerances

Food allergies involve a reaction from the immune system, which carries out a misguided attack against various food proteins. Symptoms include nausea, stomach pain, diarrhea, hives, respiratory congestion, and dizziness. For some people, food allergies trigger anaphylaxis, a life-threatening condition marked by swelling of the lips and mouth, hoarseness, difficulty breathing, wheezing, rapid heart rate, low blood pressure, confusion, and collapse.

Doctors use blood and skin tests to identify food allergies. Eight foods account for most food allergies: cow's milk; soy; wheat; eggs; peanuts; tree nuts (such as almonds, walnuts, pecans, and cashews); shellfish; and some fish. Management involves avoidance of these foods. Some food allergies such as those to milk and eggs may be outgrown. Other allergies such as those to peanuts and shellfish last a lifetime.

Unlike food allergies, food intolerances (also called food sensitivities) don't directly involve the immune system. Many times the problem stems from the digestive system's inability to digest a particular food. For example, an insufficiency of the enzyme lactase causes lactose (milk sugar) intolerance. Allergy to cow's milk, on the other hand, involves an immune system response to milk protein (casein and/or whey).

Food intolerances can cause nausea, gas, bloating, diarrhea, and headache — but no respiratory distress. Whereas a tiny amount of allergen can trigger an allergic response, it usually takes larger amounts and/or frequent exposure to elicit symptoms of intolerance.

Elimination diets can identify problem foods. The protocol usually involves eliminating the usual suspects — especially dairy and gluten-containing foods (wheat, spelt, kamut, oats, rye, barley, and malt) — from the diet for two weeks, then slowly reintroducing foods over a period of weeks while observing symptoms. Keeping a food diary provides a useful record.

Eat Beneficial Bacteria

To work properly, bodily systems such as the skin, upper respiratory tract, and digestive tract team with mutually

"Unlike food allergies, food intolerances don't directly involve the immune system. The problem stems from the body's inability to digest a particular food."

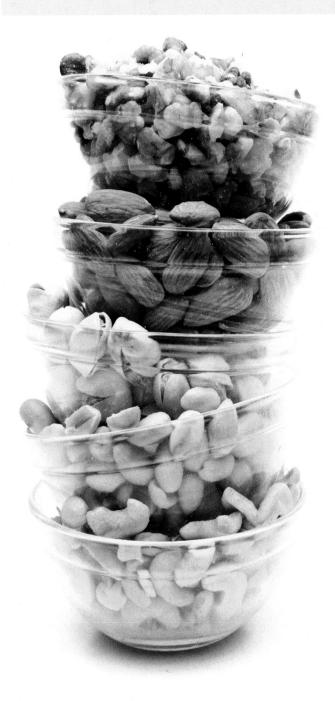

Digestive Tea

The herbs in this formula relieve cramps, bloating, and flatulence.

Ingredients

- 1 tablespoon peppermint leaves
- 1 teaspoon fennel seeds
- 1 teaspoon anise seeds
- 1 teaspoon cinnamon chips
- ½ teaspoon cardamom seeds
- 2 cups water

Directions: Combine herbs in a clean jar. Boil water; remove from heat.

Add 1 to 2 teaspoons of herb blend per cup of hot water. Cover and steep for 20 minutes. Strain and enjoy before and after meals.

Adapted from 500 Time-Tested Home Remedies and the Science Behind Them *by Linda B. White, Barbara Seeber, and Barbara Brownell Grogan; available at MotherEarthNews.com/Store.*

Tummy Rub for Pain and Bloating

This oil blend relieves intestinal upset in adults and children.

Ingredients

- 2 tablespoons olive oil
- 2 drops peppermint essential oil
- 2 drops basil essential oil
- 2 drops lavender essential oil
- 2 drops ginger essential oil

Directions: Blend ingredients in a jar.

To use, lie on your back and massage 1 to 2 teaspoons of the mixture onto your belly in a clockwise direction. Cover with a damp cloth and a hot water bottle or heating pad.

Cap and store leftovers out of reach of children. External use only.

Variation: Add 8 to 10 drops of any one of these essential oils to olive oil, then use as directed.

beneficial bacteria and fungi. Our intestines alone are home to up to 500 bacterial species — these "gut flora" outnumber our own cells by a factor of 10. They aid digestion and absorption of food, discourage colonization with disease-causing microbes, and promote immune system health.

Laboratory research suggests that gut microbes protect against autoimmune disease and inflammatory conditions. Disturbances in gut microbes have been linked with inflammatory bowel disease, obesity, and diabetes.

Probiotics are live microorganisms such as bacteria and yeast that, when consumed, offer many numerous health benefits. These come in the form of fermented foods (such as yogurt, kefir, sauerkraut, kimchi, miso, and tempeh) and even supplements.

Most of the research has focused on strains of the *Lactobacillus* species. For instance, studies have found some strains treat and prevent certain types of infectious diarrhea such as traveler's diarrhea and rotavirus infection in children. A 2010 review of 10 studies found probiotics helpful in managing IBS. Probiotic supplements and active-culture yogurt can also reduce the risk of antibiotic-associated diarrhea. Consumption of fermented dairy products such as yogurt can also relieve constipation and may reduce the risk of colon cancer.

Drink Up

Water is an essential part of our diet. Among water's many functions, adequate amounts promote regular bowel movements and prevent constipation. In fact, low fluid intake predicts constipation more reliably than low fiber. The Institute of Medicine recommends men consume an average of 3.7 liters (about 4 quarts) daily and women drink 2.7 liters (about 3 quarts) a day. However, you don't really need to track your water intake. In the absence of extreme old age (when thirst mechanisms weaken) and serious illness, thirst is a good guide.

Say 'Om'

In other words, manage stress. The intestinal tract is exquisitely sensitive to it. Stress activates our sympathetic nervous systems (fight or flight) and dials down our parasympathetic nervous systems (rest and digest). When we're stressed, blood flow to the gut decreases, saliva dries, enzyme secretion diminishes, small intestinal motility slows, and large intestinal motility speeds up. The net effect can be poor digestion, abdominal discomfort, and — with more severe stress — diarrhea.

Anxiety and stress correlate with IBS, a condition marked by abdominal pain, bloating, diarrhea, and/or constipation. Preliminary research suggests that a technique known as mindfulness-based stress reduction (MBSR), a therapy that blends yoga and mindful meditation, can ameliorate symptoms of IBS. For more information, see MindfulLivingPrograms.com.

Psychological stress also plays a role in peptic ulcers. From about 1950 through the mid-1980s, doctors thought psychological stress was the main cause of ulcers. Then blame shifted to the bacterium *Helicobacter pylori*, and the main treatment to antibiotics. Today most physicians have come to a middle ground, recognizing that stress sets the stage for and perpetuates ulcers. Other important factors include smoking, alcohol consumption, and the use of nonsteroidal anti-inflammatory drugs such as ibuprofen. ✤

Linda B. White is a Denver-based doctor, writer, and lecturer. She is the author of *Health Now: An Integrative Approach to Personal Health* and *500 Time-Tested Home Remedies and the Science Behind Them* (available at MotherEarthNews.com/Store),

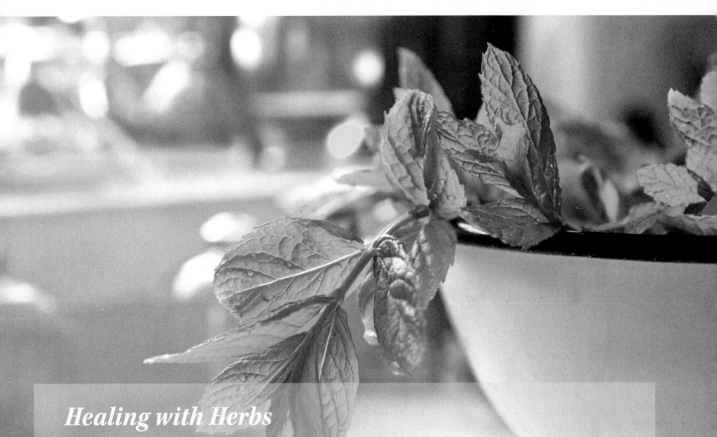

Healing with Herbs

For centuries, chefs and traditional healers alike have recommended **DIGESTIVE BITTERS** to pique the appetite and spark digestive juices. Aperitifs—alcoholic drinks taken before a meal—include "bitters," which contain herbs such as gentian, cascarilla, orange peel, cardamom, coriander, and juniper.

Another tradition for jump-starting digestion is eating a salad of **BITTER GREENS** such as endive, arugula, dandelion leaves, and radicchio, or an appetizer of **ARTICHOKE LEAVES**. Artichoke, and even more so its botanical cousin **MILK THISTLE**, also supports liver health. Artichoke leaf extract and milk thistle extract both reduce symptoms of dyspepsia (a vague term for digestive difficulties with symptoms such as nausea, heartburn, bloating, and discomfort) and irritable bowel syndrome (IBS).

FENNEL provides a host of digestive benefits. It acts as a carminative (helps expel gas), antispasmodic (to relieve painful cramping), anti-inflammatory, digestive bitter, and anti-nausea herb. After a meal, try chewing a few fennel seeds to improve digestion. You might create a tasty digestive-enhancing herbal blend of dried fennel seeds, anise seeds, and caraway seeds. To counter indigestion, chew ⅛ to ¼ teaspoon of the seed blend.

PEPPERMINT possesses antispasmodic, carminative, anti-nausea, and analgesic effects that resolve many digestive complaints. If tension has caused a headache and intestinal distress, peppermint may remedy both issues. Peppermint oil capsules have been shown safe and effective in children and adults with IBS. A combination of peppermint and caraway oil also relieves dyspepsia. Look for peppermint products that are enteric-coated, which can survive the acidic stomach then break down in the small intestine. Other mint-family herbs such as spearmint, lemon balm, catnip, and basil may also reduce painful cramping and gas.

GERMAN CHAMOMILE is a traditional digestive remedy, readily available as a tea. Slightly bitter and anti-inflammatory, this herb has been successfully combined with herbs such as peppermint and milk thistle for managing dyspepsia and IBS.

GINGER is one of my favorite medicinal and culinary plants. It's warming, anti-inflammatory, analgesic, and the best-researched herb against nausea. Studies show it counters motion sickness, post-operative nausea and vomiting, and nausea of pregnancy (pregnant women should take no more than 1 gram a day). Lab studies show ginger might prevent stomach ulcers caused by nonsteroidal anti-inflammatory drugs.

SLIPPERY ELM BARK and **MARSHMALLOW ROOT** spell relief for inflammation anywhere in the intestinal tract. You can make tea from either plant. You can also take encapsulated powdered slippery elm or mix powdered bark half and half with oats to make a soothing cereal (add minced ginger to counteract nausea and enhance taste). Tea made from red and black **RASPBERRY**—the leaves and roots—is a traditional diarrhea remedy.

A Healthy, Protected *Liver*

Take these herbs to sustain a liver that can multitask, metabolize, and maintain a smooth-running body.

By Beth Baugh and Christopher Hobbs

The liver is a truly remarkable organ that most of us fail to appreciate, considering the many vital functions it performs. As the major organ of digestion and assimilation, the liver helps to provide the nutrients that maintain health and repair diseased or damaged tissue. It also plays a crucial role in helping to eliminate toxic wastes from the body.

The Liver's Job Duties

The liver's job is to make sure the body absorbs everything it needs and dumps everything it doesn't. Its major functions include: metabolizing proteins, fats, and carbohydrates, thus providing energy and nutrients; storing vitamins, minerals, and sugar; filtering the blood and helping remove harmful chemicals and bacteria; creating bile, which breaks down fats; helping assimilate and store fat-soluble vitamins (A, E, D, and K); storing extra blood, which can be quickly released when needed; creating serum proteins, which maintain fluid balance and act as carriers; helping maintain electrolyte and water balance; creating immune substances such as gamma globulin; and breaking down and eliminating excess hormones, drugs, and exogenous chemicals.

As you can see, that is a lot of work for a single organ to do, even under the best of conditions. Unfortunately, the modern lifestyle burdens the liver with many stresses, making its job even more difficult. Adding to the insult of oily, processed foods that the liver must contend with today are human-made chemicals such as lead from gasoline, countless food additives, preservatives, pesticides, herbicides, and many other compounds.

Other common liver stressors are alcohol and recreational drugs. Furthermore, drugs administered for therapeutic purposes affect the liver as do excess hormones such as adrenaline, which our bodies create constantly in response to our fast-paced lifestyle. When stressed, the liver can store hormones for up to a year, which increases the odds for emotional imbalances such as depression and anger, as well as stress-related imbalances such as immune-system depression.

The Chinese Medicine Connection

The liver's functions include regulating the blood and emotions, according to Traditional Chinese Medicine (TCM). Because the liver controls the blood, if the menses are irregular, that points to an imbalance in the liver. Therefore, liver balance is necessary for good fertility and regular and smooth menstrual cycles, and it also plays a great role in cancer prevention. Additionally, the liver regulates bile flow, digestion, and the flow of *qi*, or vital essence. It also is thought to harmonize the emotions and help maintain a relaxed inner environment and an even-tempered disposition. TCM practitioners consider that the liver also "rules" the tendons and is manifested in the nails, so if the tendons are stiff, painful, or weak, or if the nails are pale and brittle, then it could mean the liver is failing to nourish them properly.

Significant diseases associated with the hepatic system include hepatitis, jaundice, cirrhosis, bile stagnation, and gallbladder inflammation. Liver distress calls may include: temporal headaches (ones that occur on the side of the head around the temples); emotional turbulence, including irritability for no reason, anger, depression, moodiness, and an inability to express emotions; poor digestion from bile stagnation; dry or red eyes; tenderness or pain in the liver area; and acne or psoriasis.

Relating again to TCM theory, symptoms of liver distress are divided into liver syndromes, the first of which is liver

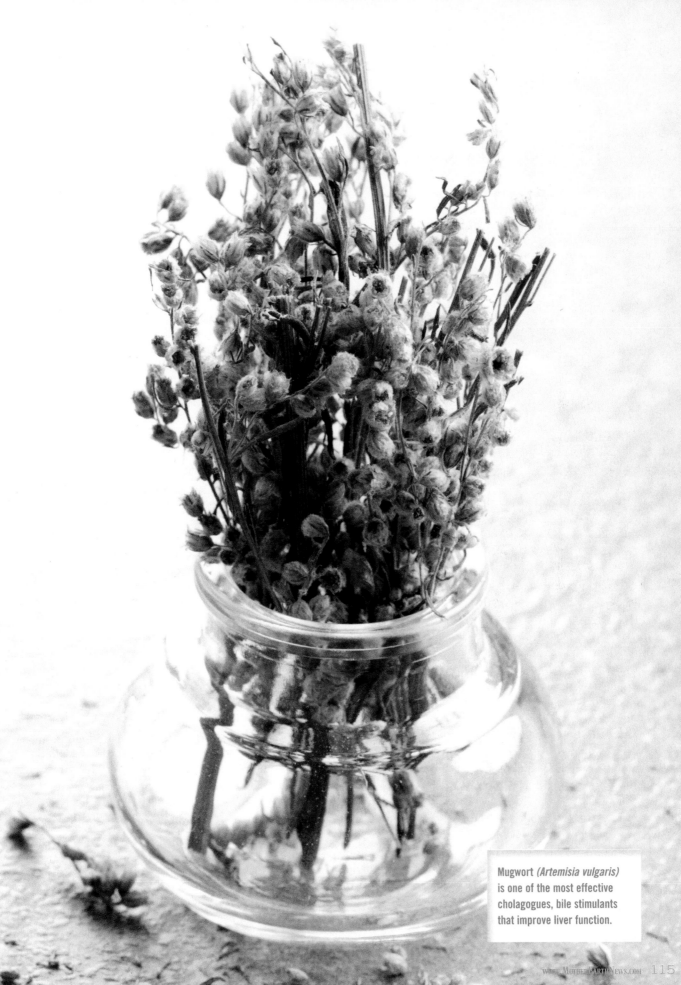

Mugwort *(Artemisia vulgaris)* is one of the most effective cholagogues, bile stimulants that improve liver function.

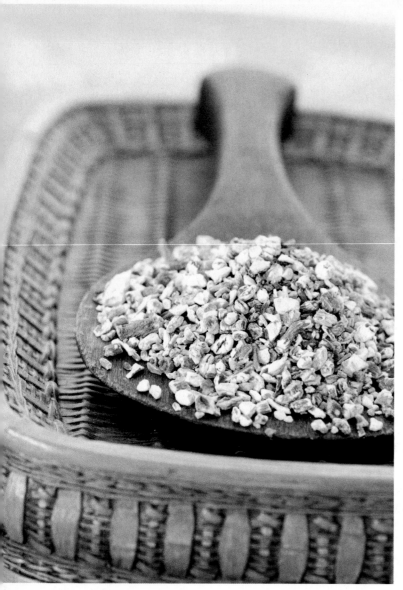

Reduce inflammation of the liver by drinking tea made with dandelion root (*Taraxacum officinale*).

America. You can make a tea of the leaves or use it as a tincture for a week or 10 days for many of the symptoms associated with liver stagnation. One other herb to try is fringetree bark (*Chionanthus virginicus*), which makes one of the best tinctures for liver stagnation. You also can purchase it in powdered form and take it in capsules, if you prefer.

Bupleurum (*Bupleurum chinense*) is a Chinese herb that is particularly effective for counteracting liver stagnation. It is an ingredient in a well-known patent formula called Shao Yao Wan that is a classic for menstrual imbalances or difficulties. It comes as little pills, and you swallow six pills three times daily around mealtimes. Taking Shao Yao Wan for 10 days may be adequate, but if you have temporal headaches or menstrual imbalances it may be necessary to take it for two to three months.

Liver heat is another common syndrome in the liver, and it involves liver inflammation or liver infection. Hepatitis is extremely common these days; not only can viral pathogens like hepatitis A, B, C, and D lead to liver inflammation, but so can bacterial and other infections. Taking certain types of toxic drugs and drinking alcohol excessively overheats the liver and can promote liver inflammation. If liver heat gets carried away, it can lead to sclerosis or scarring (cirrhosis of the liver). Symptoms of liver heat include severe temporal headaches, pain under the right rib cage, anger and irritability, itchy red eyes, and reddish color on the sides of the tongue.

To rid the body of liver heat, it is important to start using herbs as teas consistently—maybe for months or even several years—with fall-harvested dandelion root (*Taraxacum officinale*), fall-harvested burdock root (*Arctium lappa*), or gentian (*Gentiana lutea*). Gentian is one of the best cooling and regulating herbs for the liver used in both Chinese and Western medicine. American ginseng (*Panax quinquefolius*) is one of the most important herbs for people who have chronic liver conditions—cirrhosis, hepatitis, or liver heat. American ginseng is cooling and nourishing to the liver. One nice way to use American ginseng is to take a little slice of the root and put it under your tongue, suck on it, chew it, and swallow it. Because of overharvesting, don't use the wild root—use an organically cultivated variety. The ideal way to use it is to grow your own if you have some woodland space available to you.

More Liver-Loving Herbs

You can also use berberine-containing herbs for liver heat conditions. Berberine is a yellow alkaloid that has a strong cooling and bile-promoting effect on the liver. The berberine family is a great group of herbs used for various conditions. Herbs that contain berberine include Oregon grape root, which is used for skin conditions related to an overheated liver,

stagnation. When the liver is not producing enough enzymes and bile, liver stagnation will occur. After the liver produces bile, it goes to the gallbladder where it is concentrated, and then it is squirted into the small intestine to help emulsify fats. If the bile is not moving properly, you get bile stagnation, which can create a lot of health problems.

There is an entire class of herbs called cholagogues (bile stimulants) that addresses liver stagnation. Cholagogues include mugwort (*Artemisia vulgaris*) and wormwood (*Artemisia absinthium*). Of the group, we consider these two closely related herbs to be the most effective. Other useful herbs in this category are milk thistle (*Silybum marianum*), Oregon grape root (*Berberis aquifolium*), yellow dock root (*Rumex crispus*), artichoke leaf (*Cynara scolymus*), and boldo (*Peumus boldus*). These herbs are available in powdered form, tinctures, and capsules.

A member of the citrus family, boldo is considered the most important digestive liver herb in all of Mexico and South

and barberry (*Berberis vulgaris*), which grows commonly as a shrub in the eastern U.S. The root and bark of coptis (*Coptis chinensis*), a Chinese cousin to these plants, is widely used to cool the liver.

When the liver is overheated and working too hard, it starts losing its ability to produce enzymes and bile. This is called liver yin deficiency. Yin, according to TCM, is related to substances like hormones, bile, and enzymes, and when the liver is overheated and working too hard, it starts losing its ability to produce these. Dry eyes are a key sign and symptom of liver yin deficiency. Often if you can moisten, calm, and cool the liver, the problem with dry eyes will go away. This will result in more lasting improvement than putting eye drops in the eyes. Another common sign is when the sides of the tongue have no thin white coating.

The most commonly used herb for liver yin deficiency is the Chinese herb rehmannia (*Rehmannia glutinosa*). It is an ingredient in the well-known patent remedy Rehmannia 6, which commonly is used to counteract liver yin deficiency.

Creating Liver Health

While you should stay aware of liver-related symptoms, you must also work on a deeper level to balance the entire system.

Eat liver-friendly foods. Eating antioxidant-rich foods can help build and protect your liver. These include spinach, carrots, squash, broccoli, yams, tomatoes, cantaloupes, peaches, citrus fruit and juices (oranges, grapefruit), strawberries, kiwi, green peppers, raw cabbage, kale, nuts, seeds, and whole grains. Eating raw beets and beet greens also is good for nourishing the liver.

Graze on bitter herbs. Try nibbling bitter herbs—mugwort, wormwood, gentian, centaury (*Centaurium* spp.)—from the garden before meals. This is one of the finest ways of using herbs to stimulate digestion because all the energy, vitality, and healing power of the herb is right there, fresh from the garden.

Try these appetizers. Unripe fruits like plums or apples are sour and bitter, and that supposedly helps your liver digest fats. Eating a few bites before meals will have a nice cleansing and cooling action on your liver.

Sip a liver tonic tea. Make a liver tonic tea and drink a quart a day for three days. Make the tea by simmering the following herbs in a gallon of water for 20 to 30 minutes, and then strain: 3 ounces dandelion root; 3 ounces burdock root; 2 ounces schisandra fruit; 2 ounces yellow dock root; and 3 ounces orange peel. Store the tea in the refrigerator, and heat each dose before taking. Drink 1 cup in the morning and 1 cup in the evening. This is a good thing to do a few times a year.

'Flush' Your Liver Twice a Year

Liver flushes are used to stimulate elimination of wastes from the body, open and cool the liver, increase bile flow, and improve overall liver functioning. They also help purify the blood and the lymph. We recommend doing liver flushes for 10 days in the spring and again in the fall. Here's how to make a liver flush:

Mix any fresh-squeezed citrus juices together to make 1 cup of liquid. Orange and grapefruit juices are good, but always mix in some lemon or lime. The final mix should have a sour taste—the more sour, the more cleansing and activating. This mixture can be watered down to taste with spring or distilled water.

Add 1 to 2 cloves of fresh-squeezed garlic, plus a small amount of fresh ginger, which you also can squeeze through a garlic press. Garlic contains strong antioxidant properties and provides important sulfur compounds that the liver uses to build certain helpful enzymes.

Mix in 1 tablespoon high-quality olive oil. Blend in a blender (or shake well in a glass container) and drink.

Follow the liver flush with 2 cups of a cleansing herbal tea. We like the recipe for Cleansing Polari-Tea (see below). We make plenty of it and keep it in quart jars so it is readily available. **Note:** Drink the liver flush first thing in the morning. Do not eat any other food for one hour. 🌳

Beth Baugh has been the managing editor for 10 books on botanical medicine and has been involved in the herb industry for more than 30 years. Christopher Hobbs, L.Ac., is the author of *Herbal Remedies for Dummies*.

Cleansing Polari-Tea

Ingredients
- 1 teaspoon fennel seed
- 1 teaspoon fenugreek seed
- 1 teaspoon flax seed
- ½ teaspoon burdock root
- ¼ teaspoon licorice root
- 1 teaspoon peppermint leaf

Directions: Simmer fennel seed, fenugreek, flax seed, burdock, and licorice in 2½ cups of water for 20 minutes. Add peppermint and let the tea steep for an additional 10 minutes. Strain and drink. **Makes about 2 cups.**

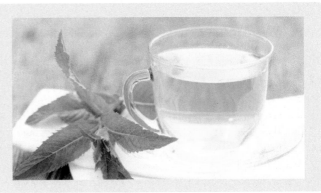

Detox with Neem

This innocuous tree is positively impacting the health of people and ecosystems around the world.

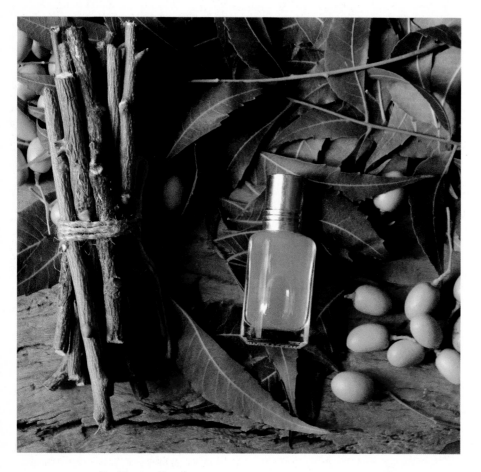

By Dawn Combs

The idea of detoxification has taken on a harsh light in our culture. It often comes with slick ads selling some sort of potion that promises to renew us after a harsh purge and a few days of fasting. I've struggled against this point of view for several years, and I suggest detoxification methods that are more balanced, even though it can be difficult to find a middle ground.

Of course, the need for detoxification is underscored by the fact that our bodies have a sophisticated system in place to do the job. One of the most important pathways through which we move the toxic byproducts of our world out of our bodies is through the liver.

I like to think of the liver as a wetland. As rivers of blood pass through it, the liver filters out the silt so that our waters will run clean as they pass through our other organs. However, the wetland can become so clogged with dirt and muck that it eventually ceases to perform this essential function. When we've overtaxed our own systems of detoxification, it becomes important to have the tools to help out.

A Dedicated Detoxifier

Neem (*Azadirachta indica*) was declared the "Tree of the 21st Century" by the United Nations, and the designation is well-deserved. I encountered the neem tree while working through my conflicting feelings about the Western fascination with harsh detox. Neem is native to India and well-known in the Ayurvedic system of healing. In India, these trees are depended upon for so much of people's daily health that they've become an expected part of the landscape, and they contain so many beneficial qualities that they're referred to as "the village pharmacy." I'd heard of neem primarily as a natural insecticide, but I wasn't aware of its use internally, as the oil in its commercial form—primarily used as a pest repellent—shouldn't be ingested.

Neem does well in dry soils and is a popular street tree in urban settings because of its hardiness, so it's been naturalized in many countries around the world. The tree is known to neutralize the acidity of soil and encourage reforestation wherever it's planted. With so many benefits to the ecosystems where it makes its home, it's not surprising to find that this tree has much to offer human health, with a strong affinity for our livers, digestion, and skin.

Neem is a balanced detoxifier whose use has been recorded in Indian medicinal wisdom as early as the 4th century

B.C. The Ayurvedic system of healing leads us to understand that detoxification isn't about harsh solutions or wild variations from our normal day-to-day routines. Instead, Ayurvedic practices focus on balance within the body's systems. This multifaceted approach suggests that the liver isn't working alone when it comes to removing toxins. In an interconnected body system, other organs will be affected by loosening chemicals, hormones, metals, and other problem substances from any major body filter. Taking care to approach detox holistically—rather than just one organ at a time—ensures we don't create a new problem elsewhere.

This is where neem shines. With its free-radical-scavenging activity, antibacterial properties, and antiviral actions, it aids the entire body in the elimination of toxins and harmful bacteria, while also strengthening the immune system. Similar to its actions neutralizing soil acidity, neem has been shown to reduce stomach acid levels and assist in the treatment of ulcers and gastrointestinal discomfort. Plus, studies reveal that *A. indica* extracts help reduce intestinal glucosidase activity and help regenerate insulin-producing cells, promising possible diabetes treatments. Also anti-inflammatory, neem is often used alongside other herbs in cooling formulas. (Learn the difference between "warming" and "cooling" Ayurvedic herbs at right.)

In neem's long history, there are few contraindications to mention beyond the need to avoid excessive use. Seek consultation for use during pregnancy and nursing, however, or if taking allopathic blood sugar control medications. Always consult a medical professional before using neem as a treatment for children.

While you can easily order neem leaves or powder from an online supplier, it's said that living near the tree itself purifies the air around it. In the U.S., only a few states, including Florida, California, and Arizona, have climates that will support neem, and few places are currently growing any measurable number of the trees. Although the rest of the country can't support the tree in an outdoor planting, that doesn't mean you can't plant your own in a pot and keep it for family use. If you decide to give growing one a try, keep in mind that this tree likes hot, dry climates and hates wet soil.

We could all benefit from a tree like neem in our Western communities to help us remember that the craze of detoxification has a foundation in good folkloric medicine, and must be viewed in a balanced manner. Including neem in your home apothecary connects you to a global village that's harvesting from this highly sustainable tree on a daily basis. It's a plant providing us solid ground in an increasingly toxic world. 🌳

> Dawn Combs is an ethnobotanist, author, co-owner of Mockingbird Meadows, and formulator of Soda Pharm syrups. Visit MockingbirdMeadows.com to learn more.

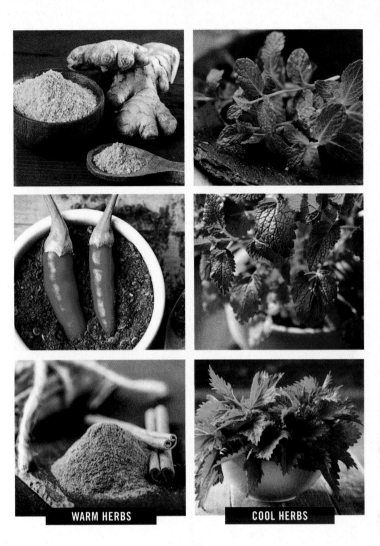

WARM HERBS

COOL HERBS

Energetics and Herbal Medicine
Why do we talk about herbs being "warming" or "cooling"?

Nearly all systems of traditional herbalism use a system of energetics for describing both health conditions and herbal medicines. It isn't hard to imagine some herbs as warm (think ginger, cayenne, and cinnamon) or cool (mint, lemon balm, and nettles). The same concepts apply to health conditions. Think of a respiratory issue and how it can feel hot and dry, such as a spastic cough, which is worse in dry air and produces thin, clear mucus, if any. Or, how it might feel cool and wet, such as a rattling, damp, less productive cough with lots of phlegm.

Although more complicated health issues can have a lot more nuance, a trained practitioner would still consider the energetics of the individual and their imbalance carefully before matching them with the most appropriate herbs. It's one of the ways herbal medicine considers the whole person, as well as the imbalance.

Bevin Clare

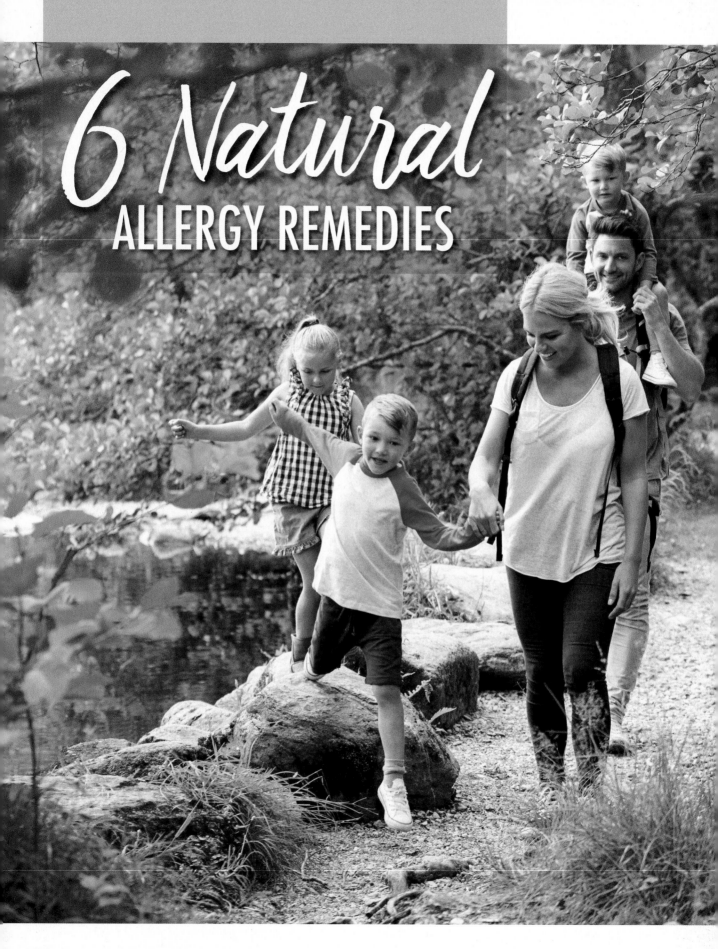

6 Natural
ALLERGY REMEDIES

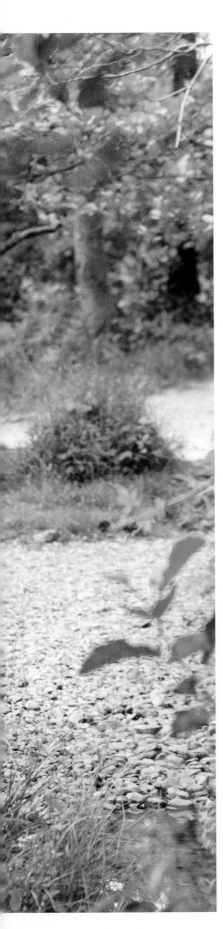

Breathe easier with medically
proven allergy treatments.

By Lynn Keiley

As soon as the golden days of summer begin to fade, thoughts often turn to the last sun-ripened tomatoes and bringing in the harvest. But if you or someone you know are among the more than 26 million Americans who suffer from seasonal allergies (or the estimated 50 million who suffer from all types of allergies), you may be focused more on pollen counts, the first freeze, and stocking up on tissues and allergy meds than on harvesting tomatoes.

Members of the sniffling, sneezing, and itching allergy demographic typically rely on numerous drugs and sprays for relief—often with mixed results. Many pharmaceutical treatments relieve sneezing and itching, but do little to treat congestion, and vice versa. In fact, at a recent meeting of the American College of Allergy, Asthma and Immunology, Dr. William E. Berger reported that nearly a third of allergy patients think their medications don't work. Plus, pharmaceutical remedies are often expensive and frequently come with unwanted side effects such as drowsiness and nasal irritation. The sedative effects of these drugs can impair driving ability and cause a mental disconnect that many users find irritating.

Annual bouts with pollen aren't just uncomfortable, they also take a toll on mental well-being. Studies have shown that during ragweed season, allergy sufferers often experience a general sense of fatigue—especially mental fatigue—and are more prone to feelings of sadness. People who suffer from allergies also are up to 14 times more likely to experience migraine headaches than those who don't have allergies.

Given these statistics, you might want to pull the covers over your head and wait until the whole season blows over. But it is possible to step outdoors safely without first loading up on allergy medications, even when ragweed is in full bloom.

Here are several natural alternatives that are medically proven to help control allergies and help you breathe easier, even when pollen counts are at their worst.

Understanding Allergies

When you understand what's happening during allergy attacks, treating them naturally seems like plain common sense. First, picture a grain of pollen—it looks something like a spiny sea urchin (see Page 122). Now imagine this prickly invader entering your nasal passages and latching onto soft mucous membranes. These mucous membranes line our bronchial and nasal passages and contain immune cells (called mast cells), which are loaded with histamines. Receptors sit on top of these mast cells, and when an allergen trigger such as pollen, mold, or pet dander lands on top of the receptor, it alerts the mast cells, which respond by releasing histamine and other chemicals. The histamine initiates a series of reactions designed to help the body get rid of the intruder, including sneezing, watery eyes, and itching. For some people, particularly

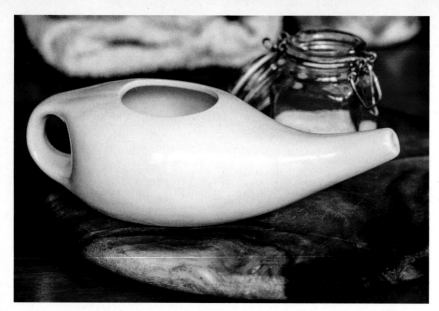

To soothe allergy attacks, consider using neti pots to flush out your nose. These pots are a mild and effective way to treat seasonal allergies.

mix ¼ to ½ teaspoon of noniodized table salt into 1 cup of lukewarm water, and pour it into the pot. (You can adjust the amount of salt, depending on what feels most comfortable.) Lean over a sink with your head slightly cocked to one side, then put the spout of the neti into one nostril and allow the water to drain out the other nostril. Use about half of the solution, then repeat on the other side, tilting your head the opposite way. Gently blow out each nostril to clear them completely. Neti pots are widely available online and at natural food stores. Use your pot about twice a day during allergy season, especially in the morning and after spending time outdoors. You also can use a neti pot before bed to prevent snoring caused by allergies and promote optimal overnight breathing.

those with asthma, this reaction may also include swelling in the bronchial tubes that makes it difficult to breathe.

Natural Remedies

Most allergy medications attempt to treat the symptoms your body instigates to get rid of the allergen. But doesn't it make more sense to shore up your defenses before your body goes into attack mode? Many of the natural remedies discussed below are designed to prevent a reaction before it occurs.

A few minor lifestyle changes also can go a long way toward keeping symptoms under control. For example:

• Avoid using window fans to cool rooms because they can pull pollen indoors.

• Keep windows closed when driving, using the air conditioner if necessary, to avoid allergens.

• Limit your time outdoors when ragweed pollen counts are highest—from mid-August until the first frost.

Here are more things that can help head off allergies before they start, as well as some drug-free ways to treat symptoms when they do arise.

Neti Pots. What could be simpler than rinsing away allergens with saltwater? Neti pots, small vessels shaped like Aladdin's lamp, have been used in India for thousands of years to flush the sinuses and keep them clear. It's an idea that takes some getting used to for most Westerners, but it's a bit like using nasal spray. A little douse of saltwater can rinse away those prickly pollen grains and help treat allergies and other forms of sinus congestion.

An Italian study published in the *International Archives of Allergy and Immunology* found that nasal flushing was a mild and effective way to treat seasonal allergies in children, and markedly reduced their use of antihistamines.

You could simply use your cupped hand instead of a neti pot to rinse sinuses, but netis are inexpensive, and many people find them much easier to use. To flush your sinuses,

Quercetin. A natural plant-derived compound called a bioflavonoid, quercetin helps stabilize mast cells and prevents them from releasing histamine. Quercetin also is a natural antioxidant that helps mop up molecules called free radicals that cause cell damage, which can lead to cancer. Citrus fruits, onions, apples, parsley, tea, tomatoes, broccoli, lettuce, and wine are naturally high in quercetin, but allergy sufferers will most likely need to use supplements to build up enough of this compound to prevent attacks. The recommended dosage is about 1,000 mg a day, taken between meals. It's best to start treatment six weeks before allergy season. Those with liver disease shouldn't use quercetin, so please consult your doctor before using this or any other supplement—especially if you are pregnant or nursing.

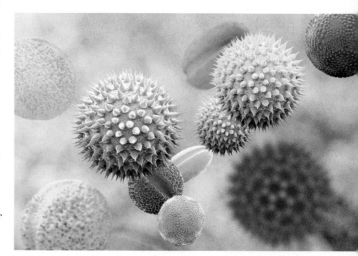

When pollen grains, such as these from ragweed, enter your nasal passages and lodge onto mucous membranes, your body responds by producing histamine, which can cause allergy symptoms such as sneezing, itching, and watery eyes.

Allergy-Fighting Foods. A German study, published in the journal *Allergy*, found that participants who ate foods rich in omega-3 fatty acids were less likely to suffer allergy symptoms than those who didn't regularly eat these foods. Omega-3s help fight inflammation and can be found in cold-water fish, walnuts, and flax seed oil, as well as grass-fed meat and eggs.

To help keep airways clear when pollen counts are high, add a dash of horseradish, chili peppers, or hot mustard to your food—all act as natural, temporary decongestants. It's also a good idea to avoid foods that you're slightly allergic to until the air clears. Fighting off allergies can render the body hypersensitive to those foods, causing more severe reactions than usual.

Stinging Nettle. If you decide you need an antihistamine but want a natural option, stinging nettle (*Urtica dioica*) behaves in much the same way as many of the drugs sold to treat allergies, but without the unwanted side effects of dry mouth and drowsiness. Nettle actually inhibits the body's ability to produce histamine. It's a common weed in many parts of the U.S., but the most practical medicinal form is a freeze-dried extract of the leaves sold in capsules. Studies have shown that taking about 300 mg daily will offer relief for most people, although the effects may last only a few hours. You also can make your own tinctures or teas with stinging nettle. (Contact with the stinging hairs on fresh nettle can cause skin inflammation, so wear protective gloves when handling it.)

Butterbur. Derived from a common weed in Europe, butterbur (*Petasites hybridus*) is another alternative to antihistamines, though it may be hard to find in the U.S. In the days before refrigeration, its broad, floppy leaves were used to wrap butter during warm spells, hence the name butterbur. A Swiss study, published in *British Journal of Medicine*, found that butterbur was as effective as the drug cetirizine, the active ingredient in Zyrtec. Even though cetirizine is supposed to be a nonsedative antihistamine, researchers reported that it did cause drowsiness, though butterbur did not. Participants in the study took 32 milligrams of butterbur a day, divided into four doses. A word of caution though—butterbur is in the same family as ragweed, so it could worsen allergy symptoms in some cases. Effects of taking butterbur over a long period of time also are unknown.

Sublingual Immunotherapy. Specific immunotherapy, otherwise known as allergy shots, has been used widely to inject patients with diluted doses of certain allergens to help build immunity over time. However, allergy shots can take three to five years to be effective, and a small percentage of

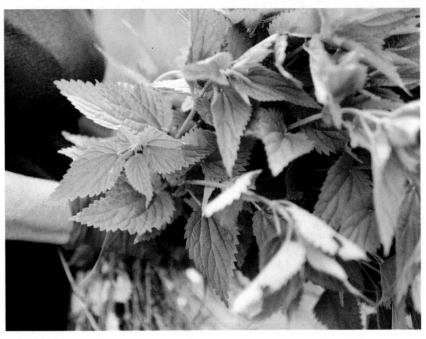

Freeze-dried extract from the leaves of stinging nettle works like an over-the-counter antihistamine, but without the unwanted side effects of dry mouth and drowsiness.

people suffer severe reactions to this treatment. Though it remains popular in some parts of the world, the practice fell out of favor in the United Kingdom during the late 1980s, when strict limitations were imposed after several adverse reactions occurred.

New studies have found a gentler way to acclimate the body to pollen and other allergens. The latest form of this therapy is called sublingual immunotherapy (SLIT), which has been used for the past 20 years in Europe. In SLIT treatments, patients put drops of a very small dose of the allergen (initially a 1:1,000 dilution) under the tongue for two minutes, then swallow. The daily therapy begins before peak pollen season for seasonal allergy sufferers, but also can be used to treat year-round allergies, though treatment must be specific to the type of allergen.

A recent study in the United Kingdom found that patients who used SLIT for two years were nearly seven times less likely to suffer runny noses, and almost three times less likely to experience sneezing, than those who took a placebo. Before considering SLIT therapy, check with your doctor and insurance provider (as it is not covered by most insurances). The only FDA-approved sublingual therapy is tablets. Allergy drops are not FDA-approved and are off-label in the U.S., according to the American College of Allergy, Asthma & Immunology.

Whether you suffer from seasonal or ongoing allergies, these natural remedies should let you get out there and harvest those late tomatoes! ❧

Lynn Keiley, a freelance writer from Pennsylvania, keeps springtime allergies at bay with the use of her trusty neti pot.

HEAL
the Skin You're In

Find herbal relief
for skin diseases
including eczema,
psoriasis, and rosacea.

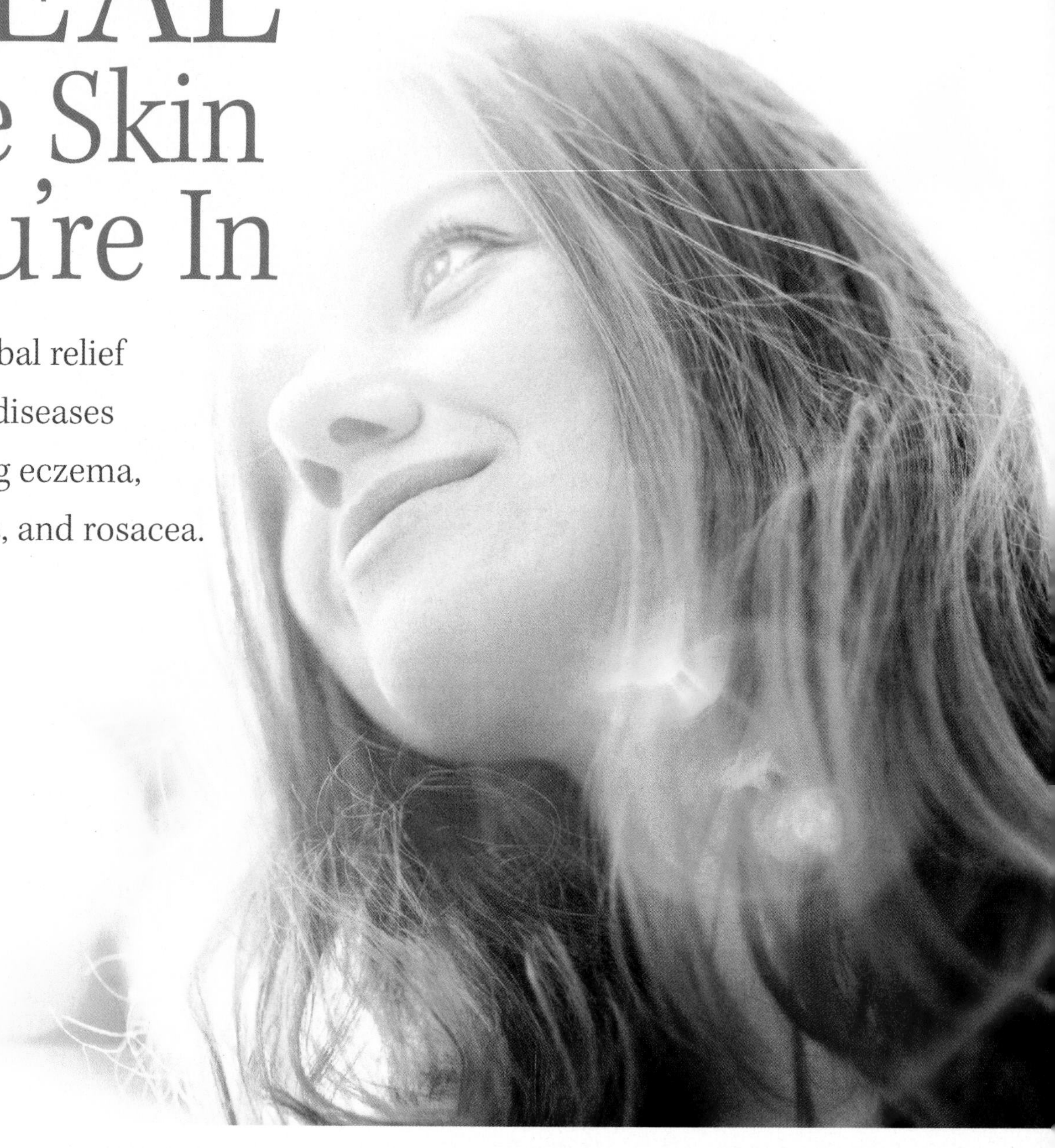

By Kim Erickson

Achieving healthy, glowing skin is an attainable dream for many. But for the millions of people who suffer from eczema, psoriasis, or rosacea, the redness, scaling, sores, and incessant itching that mark these chronic skin conditions can lead to a lifetime of discomfort and embarrassment. Conventional treatments aren't always effective and often rely on antibiotics and topical steroids that can thin the skin, weaken an already delicate immune system, and damage the liver. Fortunately Mother Nature has a number of safe, effective tricks up her sleeve to help control these troubling diseases.

Calming Eczema

Are you the sensitive type? If your skin seems to react to everything from stress to perfume, you may have eczema. Also known as dermatitis in medical-speak, eczema is actually a group of skin conditions that affects one in every 12 American adults. Caused by genetic factors, stress, an allergic reaction, or yeast growths, eczema often appears as red, itchy, inflamed, scaly, or even crusty, oozing patches of skin. People with thin, dry skin are more susceptible.

Luckily there are a number of natural steps you can take to ease eczema. First, it's important to do some sleuthing to find out what causes flare-ups. For some people, it can be as simple as a change in climate. For others, stress or illness can worsen the disease.

Certain foods, fabrics, or the chemicals commonly used in cosmetics and cleaning products can also make symptoms worse. If you can pinpoint what makes your skin rage, take whatever steps you can to avoid the offender.

Botanicals can help heal the outbreaks that do occur. According to naturopathic doctor Tori Hudson, author of the *Women's Encyclopedia of Natural Medicine*, evening primrose oil (*Oenothera biennis*), a rich source of gamma linolenic acid (GLA), can help your skin retain moisture and may protect it from environmental oxidative damage. One recent study by Korean researchers at Inha University found that evening primrose oil not only reduces skin lesions and itching, it also helps modulate the immune system.

"There have been many scientific studies using GLA with excellent benefits in improving the symptoms of eczema," Hudson says. She recommends supplementing the diet with 500 to 3,000 mg of evening primrose oil daily.

Packed with polyphenols, oolong tea (partially fermented *Camellia sinensis*) can also soothe stubborn eczema. Researchers from the Shiga University School of Medical Science in Japan discovered this when patients undergoing treatment for their eczema began drinking oolong tea three times a day. Their skin health improved in as little as one week. After a month, 65 percent of the 118 participants showed significant improvement.

"Herbs are particularly helpful when applied topically," holistic cosmetologist Denise Santamarina says. Santamarina is the owner of Natural Nouveaux, a nontoxic salon and day spa in Las Vegas. Chamomile (*Matricaria chamomilla*), aloe (*Aloe vera*), and witch hazel (*Hamamelis virginiana*) are her top picks for eczema because of their ability to reduce inflammation.

Fenugreek (*Trigonella foenum-graecum*) is recommended by the German Commission E to treat eczema-related inflammation. While some eczema ointments contain fenugreek, you can make your own poultice by mixing the powdered seed with enough hot water to form a thin paste. Dip a clean cotton cloth in the paste and apply to the affected area. Leave on for five to 10 minutes, rinse with tepid water, and pat dry.

Moisturizers containing emollient herbs such as marshmallow (*Althaea officinalis*) can help prevent dryness. And calendula (*Calendula officinalis*) can speed the healing of broken skin. According to renowned herbalist James A. Duke, research on calendula shows this herb is antibacterial, antifungal, anti-inflammatory, and antiviral. And because of the powerful broad-spectrum antimicrobial activity of tea tree (*Melaleuca alternifolia*) oil, this botanical is being looked at for its ability to treat eczema caused by *Candida albicans* and allergic hypersensitivity.

Perhaps the most frustrating symptom of eczema is the constant, sometimes

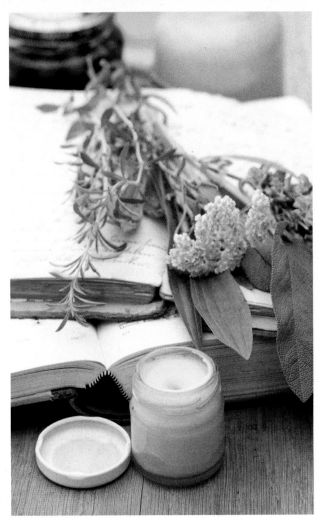

Herbs are especially helpful to irritated skin when applied topically. Use ointments made with chamomile, aloe, or witch hazel.

severe, itching that can leave you raw and bleeding. Cnidium (*Cnidium monnieri*) has been valued by practitioners of Asian folk medicine for centuries because of its antibacterial and astringent effects. New research by the Institute of Natural Medicine in Toyama, Japan, has found that this herb is also a potent antipruritic (itch-reliever) when used topically. The herb is available in many Asian markets, and you can make an effective anti-itch poultice by mixing ground cnidium seeds with water. There is still not enough safety information about cnidium, so pregnant and breast-feeding women should not use it.

Psoriasis Secrets

For the nearly 5 million Americans who suffer from psoriasis, it's almost as if their skin is set on fast-forward. Normally, skin cells go from birth to death in about 28 days, but with psoriasis, skin cells complete the whole process in a mere three to four days. As a result, affected areas develop thick, red patches of skin covered with flaky, silvery scales. In severe cases, pus-filled blisters form on the palms of the hands or soles of the feet, and the nails may become pitted and discolored. While psoriasis tends to be inherited, its cause is open to speculation. Many researchers believe it's an autoimmune disorder. Others think it's a defect in the body's natural detoxification process. Still others point to nutritional causes and stress. Common triggers may include injury to the skin, some infections, and reaction to certain drugs. One thing is certain: There is no known cure. But you can control the severity of the disease.

For some psoriasis sufferers, dietary changes may be beneficial. Turkish researchers found that people with psoriasis have low levels of key antioxidant vitamins A, C, and E. Eating plenty of fruits and vegetables will ensure you're getting adequate amounts of antioxidants to support healthy skin. Selenium also plays an important role

in the disease. One case-controlled study of 59 psoriasis patients and 38 patients without the disease discovered that those with psoriasis were deficient in selenium. Selenium can be found in whole grains, garlic, onions, broccoli, tomatoes, and Swiss chard. A diet rich in omega-3 essential fatty acids can also tame the inflammation that accompanies psoriasis. Fish and flax seeds are excellent sources.

Sunlight can help send psoriasis packing—at least temporarily. In fact, some doctors employ prescription ultraviolet light boxes combined with certain drugs that increase sun sensitivity. But this "new" treatment is actually thousands of years old, Duke says.

Known as heliotherapy or light ther-

apy, ancient Egyptians rubbed red, scaly skin with plants containing compounds called psoralens and then sat in the sun. According to Duke, psoralen-rich plants, including angelica (*Angelica archangelica*), carrots, celery, citrus fruits, fennel (*Foeniculum vulgare*), figs, lovage (*Levisticum officinale*), and thyme (*Thymus vulgaris*), can provide a safer, gentler way to boost the healing power of the sun.

For a pleasant treatment, Duke suggests trying his Psoriaphobic Citrus Juice. "Simply toss a mixture of citrus fruits, a carrot, and a celery stalk into your juicer," he says. Once you've finished drinking this tasty treatment, go out into the sun for some homemade heliotherapy. Long-term exposure to the sun can increase your risk of skin cancer, so practice this therapy with caution.

Even without the benefit of the sun, herbs play a key role in controlling psoriasis. Scientists from London's King's College found that gotu kola (*Centella asiatica*) was as effective at slowing the rampant production of skin cells as a synthetic anti-psoriatic treatment. Another study found that an ointment containing Oregon grape (*Berberis aquifolium*) also helped stop overactive cell production. What's more, earlier research shows that Oregon grape can boost the skin's immune response and soothe moderate psoriasis by reducing inflammation and itching.

Recent studies have also found that fumitory (*Fumaria officinalis*) can help patients with severe psoriasis. Although how this particular botanical works is a topic of hot debate, some researchers believe that the fumaric acid esters in the herb modulate the T-cell response. Duke recommends brewing a strong tea of the herb and applying it to the affected area with a cotton ball three times daily.

When it comes to caring for psoriatic skin, Santamarina suggests dry brushing the skin with a natural-bristle brush to exfoliate the build-up of dead skin cells. (This may be painful for some psoriasis sufferers; don't use this treatment if it hurts.)

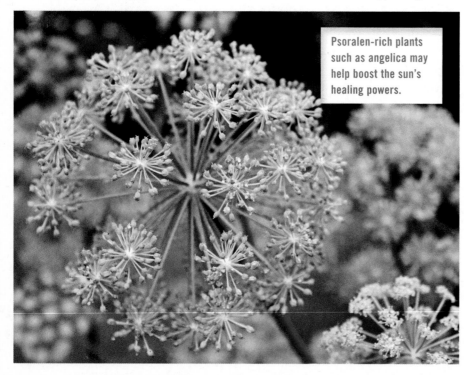

Psoralen-rich plants such as angelica may help boost the sun's healing powers.

"Begin at your feet and work your way up over your legs, torso, and arms using smooth, upward strokes," she says. "Then hop in the shower to wash all of the dead skin away."

For an even more effective treatment, follow your dry brushing with a bath containing Dead Sea salts. High in magnesium, potassium, calcium, and iodine, a double-blind controlled study of 23 patients by Israeli researchers found that Dead Sea salts significantly reduced psoriasis symptoms.

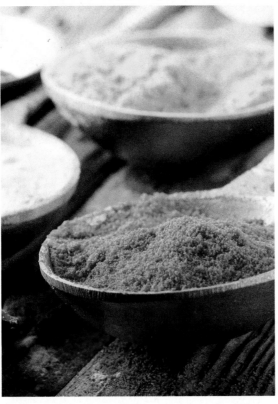
Benefit from turmeric's anti-inflammatory properties with a homemade paste: 1 part turmeric powder, 4 parts water.

War of the Rosacea

When the blush of youth turns into an embarrassing redness that never seems to go away, you may be suffering from rosacea. Rosacea is a disease that can make even teetotalers look like long-time alcoholics. It's an unglamorous problem that affects 13 million Americans, including former President Bill Clinton.

Although no one is quite sure what causes rosacea, some studies have found a connection between this skin condition and the ulcer bug, Helicobacter pylori. Others point to Demodex folliculorum, a microscopic mite that lives on dead skin cells. Whatever the cause, rosacea is a chronic condition that first appears as excessive flushing across the cheeks, chin, nose, and forehead. Eventually, this redness is accompanied by small, unsightly blood vessels. In many people, rosacea doesn't end with flushing and blushing; it can lead to inflammation and acne-like bumps and pimples.

Any number of factors can bring on the redness. Cheese, chocolate, soy sauce, citrus fruits, spicy foods, and alcohol can make rosacea worse, as can hot tea, coffee, or soups. Stress can also trigger a flare-up. And because heat can make rosacea worse, it's wise to avoid saunas, hot baths, and excessively warm environments. Even exercise can be your enemy, especially workouts that raise body temperature and increase blood flow to the face.

"You have to be especially careful when it comes to using cosmetics and skin-care products if you have rosacea," Santamarina says. "Avoid anything that contains alcohol or acetone. And if a product causes redness or stinging, stop using it." If you do become overheated or even encounter a product that worsens the disease, soak a washcloth in ice water spiked with a few drops of lavender (*Lavandula angustifolia*) essential oil. Then wring out the cloth and place it over your face for about two or three minutes.

While there is a scientific gap when it comes to herbal therapies for rosacea, folk remedies abound. Tonic herbs such as burdock (*Arctium lappa*) and yellow dock (*Rumex crispus*) have been used internally for years because of their cleansing properties. Some herbalists also recommend applying herbal waters of skin-friendly botanicals like Roman chamomile (*Chamaemelum nobile*) or rose (*Rosa* spp.).

Serious Skin Care

Whether you have rosacea, psoriasis, or eczema, caring for this trio of conditions can leave those afflicted in a complexion conundrum. Holistic cosmetologist Denise Santamarina recommends forgetting everything you've learned about the "right" way to care for your skin. Whether you have eczema, psoriasis, or rosacea, she advises washing your face with a nonabrasive herbal cleanser designed for sensitive skin and lukewarm (not hot) water.

Blot, don't rub, your face with a thick-pile cotton towel and wait until your face is completely dry before applying any other skin-care products. "If you suffer from rosacea, never, ever exfoliate," she warns. But for her clients with eczema or psoriasis, she often recommends using either plain oatmeal or cornmeal to clean away bacteria and accumulated skin cells.

When it comes to makeup, Santamarina says covering your condition with a heavy layer of traditional cosmetics can make matters worse. "If you must wear makeup, opt for one made from pure minerals instead of oils or harsh chemicals."

Recently, scientists at King George's Medical College in Lucknow, India, gave a nod to the effectiveness of traditional remedies — they acknowledged the success Ayurvedic practitioners have had in treating chronic skin diseases with anti-inflammatory herbs such as turmeric (*Curcuma longa*) and neem (*Azadirachta indica*). But you don't need to travel to India to benefit from these ancient therapies. You can find turmeric powder, a mild-tasting ingredient in curry spice, in supermarkets or in capsule form at your local health-food store. Topical neem oil is also becoming a staple at health-food stores and can even be found in some skin- and hair-care products. 🌿

Kim Erickson is the author of *Drop Dead Gorgeous: Protecting Yourself from the Hidden Dangers of Cosmetics*.

Marvelous Myrrh

A little myrrh essential oil goes a long way in rejuvenating skin, among other skin-healing benefits.

By Stephanie Tourles

Myrrh—an aromatic, rich, precious resin—was widely used in ancient times throughout the Middle East (especially in Egypt) for incense, perfumery, medicine, and as a preservation ingredient in the embalming process. It was particularly prized as a remedial aid for infections of the respiratory tract, mouth, and skin; and as a digestive stimulant. Myrrh was also one of the three gifts said to have been brought by the three wise men to the baby Jesus to support a state of grace and preserve divine essence. The name myrrh derives from the Arabic *murr*, meaning "bitter."

Myrrh (*Commiphora myrrha*) essential oil is valued for many of the same uses as the resin. Known for its rejuvenating and revitalizing effects on the skin, it is often used in natural anti-aging products to delay wrinkling and improve the skin's texture and tone. I swear by myrrh essential oil's "youthifying" effects and often add a few drops to my facial oils and creams. A little goes a long way. It also successfully promotes the healing of all manner of minor wounds, inflamed skin conditions (such as weeping eczema and psoriasis, hemorrhoids, and acne), and environmentally damaged, dry, chapped, cracked skin.

Myrrh essential oil has a superb reputation as a remedy for inflammatory and infectious conditions of the mouth and throat (bleeding gums, gingivitis, ulcers, bad breath, pyor-

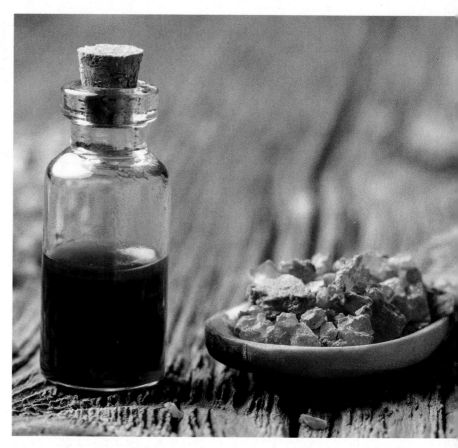

rhea, receding gums, thrush, general sore throat, laryngitis, and tonsillitis). It also serves as a most useful respiratory antiseptic with drying and purifying properties that help alleviate infection and loosen and expectorate mucus during cases of bronchitis, sinusitis, asthma, coughs, and colds.

From Herb to Oil

The scrubby, thorny myrrh tree has knotted branches, small three-part leaves, and white flowers. When pierced or incised, the trunk and larger limbs yield a pale-yellow liquid

that hardens into the reddish-brown drops known as myrrh or myrrh gum resin. These are dried to be distilled into essential oil or used as incense.

The tree is native to the Middle East, northeast Africa, and southwest Asia, though its growing range has been extended by cultivation. The essential oil is primarily distilled in Somalia, Ethiopia, and Sudan.

Myrrh essential oil is produced by steam distillation of the crude gum oleoresin. A lovely, sweeter carbon dioxide is also produced in lesser quantity, as is a resinoid and resin absolute. It is an oily, pale yellow-to-amber, viscous liquid with a rather unique odor: warm, sweet-balsamic, slightly spicy-medicinal-astringent, smoky-musty.

The myrrh tree belongs to the same plant family (Burseraceae) as frankincense (*Boswellia carteri*, *B. sacra*, *B. frereana*, and multiple other *Boswellia* species). Both species grow slowly in arid climates, and due to the popularity of their resins, the wild trees cannot sustainably produce enough to fill the global demand. They are both considered vulnerable and near-threatened. I ask that you use the beloved myrrh and frankincense products judiciously and sparingly. Frankincense and myrrh are now being cultivated to help satisfy demand, but as I said, their growth is very slow.

Myrrh tones and tightens skin tissue and is highly antibacterial; astringent; anti-inflammatory; the best remedy for mouth, gum, and throat irritations and infections; a powerful respiratory antiseptic and expectorant; stimulating; and warming.

It also strengthens and fortifies the emotions as it is grounding and centering to the mind.

Safety Data & Usage Information

Myrrh is generally nonirritating and nonsensitizing. Avoid use during pregnancy, while breastfeeding, and with children under 2 years of age.

Always dilute essential oils properly—according to age, health, medication intake, and skin condition—prior to application.

The recipe at right highlights the therapeutic nature of myrrh essential oil with regard to its benefits for oral health. Combined with peppermint essential oil, it works like a charm. 🌿

Stephanie Tourles has been practicing and teaching healthy living for more than 25 years. She is a licensed holistic esthetician and a certified aromatherapist.

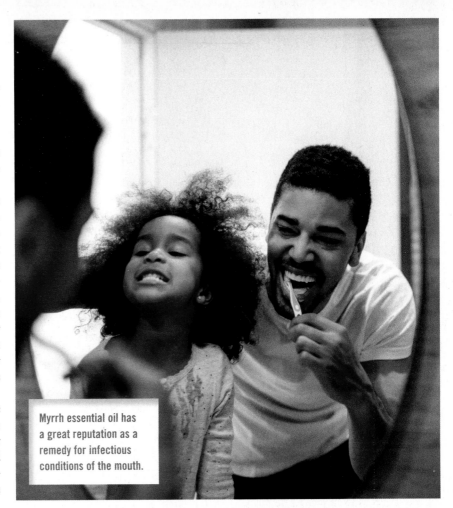

Myrrh essential oil has a great reputation as a remedy for infectious conditions of the mouth.

Soothing Myrrh-Mint Mouthwash & Gargle

With a combination of warm, resinous notes and stimulating, sharp mint, this bracing, mouth-tingling blend offers antibacterial, astringent, analgesic, and anti-inflammatory properties that help tone and tighten gum tissue, neutralize bad breath, soothe a sore throat, relieve laryngitis, and aid in alleviating mouth ulcers and inflamed gums. It is tasty and effective. **Note:** This recipe is safe for folks 12 years of age and older. **Makes one single use.**

Ingredients
- 1 drop myrrh (*Commiphora myrrha*) essential oil
- 1 drop peppermint (*Mentha piperita*) essential oil
- ¼ teaspoon sea salt
- ¼ cup purified water, hot or tepid (hot water is more soothing for sore throats and laryngitis)

Directions: Combine drops of myrrh and peppermint essential oils with sea salt in a small mug. Pour in water and stir to blend. Use immediately.

To use, first rinse your mouth thoroughly with plain water, then gargle and swish with half of the mouthwash for up to 30 seconds (or for as long as you can tolerate). Spit it out in the sink (do not swallow). Repeat with remaining mouthwash. If you are suffering from a sore throat or laryngitis, mouth ulcers, bleeding gums, or pyorrhea, repeat several times per day until the condition improves, making a new batch each time.

Recipe excerpted from Stephanie Tourles' Essential Oils: A Beginner's Guide, *(©2018 by Stephanie Tourles). Used with permission from Storey Publishing.*

The Value of Geranium

Geranium essential oil is a soothing astringent, making it an excellent choice for treating eczema and psoriasis.

By Stephanie Tourles

This highly aromatic plant, long adored for the delicious complexity of its bouquet, has been much used by the perfume industry for hundreds of years. Seventeenth-century Europeans loved it so much that they developed hundreds of hybrids. Geranium leaves make a soothing rose-flavored tea and are prized for their use in making a fragrant body wash, hydrosol, natural deodorant, and effective insect repellent. They can also be used to promote healing for a broad range of conditions, from dysentery and cholera to hemorrhoids and infections of the skin.

As a soothing astringent, geranium (*Pelargonium graveolens*; *P. ×asperum*) essential oil tones and tightens the skin and astringes excess moisture, making it an excellent choice for weeping eczema, psoriasis, edema, hemorrhoids, and excessive perspiration of underarms and feet. Considered a "beautifying oil," it benefits the health of both the skin and scalp by balancing sebum (oil) production in all skin types. With its parasiticidal properties, it is also useful in blends formulated to combat ringworm, lice, nail fungus, and athlete's foot.

For those with impaired circulation or vascular disorders, such as Raynaud's disease, couperose skin (skin exhibiting diffuse redness due to dilated capillaries), or varicose and spider veins, geranium essential oil, in addition to other oils such as cypress (*Cupressus sempervirens*) and ginger (*Zingiber officinale*), is a useful adjunct to assist with regulation of blood flow.

Sometimes called "the woman's oil," geranium essential oil is indeed a special gift for women because of its positive regulatory actions upon the hormones secreted by the adrenal cortex. This makes it a valuable remedy for problems caused by fluctuating hormone levels, including PMS, engorged and/or painful breasts, and menopausal symptoms such as hot flashes and vaginal dryness.

Geranium Oil or Rose Oil?

Geranium essential oil is sometimes confused with rose (*Rosa damascena*) essential oil, due to its rose-like scent

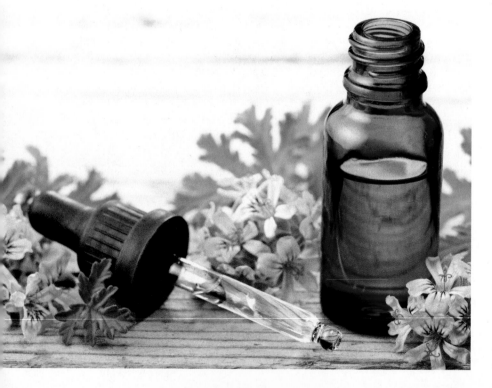

and the fact that it's occasionally labeled "rose geranium." In fact, geranium oil is frequently used to adulterate and extend real rose oil, and it is the starting point in the manufacture of synthetic rose oil.

A native of South Africa, this tender perennial fuzzy shrub has pointed leaves and clusters of small pink, violet, red, or white flowers. The entire plant is aromatic. The genus name *Pelargonium* derives from the Greek *pelargos*, "stork," in reference to the herb's long, bill-like seeds. More than 250 varieties of scented geraniums are cultivated all over the world. *P. graveolens* is the name most often found on commercial essential oil labels, although it is unlikely to be the true botanical source.

The leaves, green stems, and flowers are harvested at the start of the flowering period and steam-distilled to produce the clear, slightly greenish essential oil. As I mentioned earlier, the scent, though lovely, can be a bit heavy and likes to cling and linger, so follow any recipes to the letter and use a light hand if adding to your diffuser — perhaps starting with just one drop.

When purchasing geranium essential oil, you may have a choice between Egyptian, Chinese, and Bourbon varieties. The Egyptian, which tends to be the least expensive, has a less-sweet, grassy-rose aroma. The Chinese smells like typical geranium, being rosy-earthy-green. The Bourbon is the cream of the crop, with an exquisitely clean and sweet scent, but it is also the most expensive. They all work equally well in my recipes; it's just a matter of taste and budget.

"Balancing" is the best way to describe this oil. It seems to bestow upon you what you need. It is gently refreshing, uplifting, calming, grounding, and centering, yet not sedating. The aroma encourages feelings of peace and harmony,

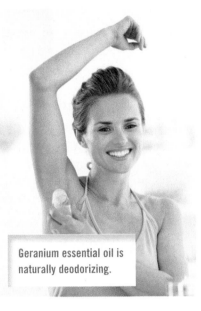
Geranium essential oil is naturally deodorizing.

while uncluttering a chaotic mind. It is useful for treating depression, nervous tension, anxiety, and restlessness, and it's a wonderful choice for those moving through a stressful, symptomatic menopause.

It is a gentle astringent and diuretic, good for water retention/edema; antibacterial and antifungal; a mild anti-inflammatory and moderate circulatory stimulant; deodorizing; promotes wound healing; cooling; emotionally and physically balancing; and a valuable insect repellent and parasiticide.

Generally considered nontoxic, nonirritating, and nonsensitizing, geranium may cause contact dermatitis in hypersensitive individuals. Always dilute essential oils properly — according to age, health, medication intake, and skin condition — prior to application.

The recipe at right highlights the therapeutic nature of geranium essential oil with regard to its deodorizing properties. Works like a charm. 🌿

Stephanie Tourles has been practicing and teaching healthy living for more than 25 years. She is a licensed holistic esthetician and a certified aromatherapist.

Herbal Fresh Deodorant Spray

The most important action of any deodorant is to minimize the proliferation of odor-causing bacteria, and this formula, with its delightful aroma, does it amazingly well, sans synthetic fragrance and questionable ingredients. Keep a small bottle with a few cotton pads handy for when you need to freshen up a bit. It's wonderful as a foot deodorizer, too. **Note:** This recipe is safe for people 6 years of age and older. **Makes 8-ounces.**

Ingredients
- 1 cup unflavored vodka (80-proof) or commercially prepared witch hazel
- ½ teaspoon vegetable glycerin
- 16 drops geranium (*Pelargonium graveolens*; *P. ×asperum*) essential oil
- 12 drops rosemary (*Rosmarinus officinalis* chemotype verbenon) essential oil
- 12 drops tea tree (*Melaleuca alternifolia*) essential oil
- 8 drops lemon (*Citrus limon*) essential oil
- One 8-ounce plastic or dark glass spritzer bottle

Directions: Pour vodka (or witch hazel) into bottle. Add glycerin, then geranium, rosemary, tea tree, and lemon essential oils. Screw the top on the bottle and shake vigorously to blend — expect essential oils to separate out and float to the top in about 5 minutes, as that's normal. Label the bottle and allow the spray to synergize for at least 1 hour. Store at room temperature, away from heat and light; use within 1 year.

To use, shake well and use immediately. Spray onto clean, dry underarms and/or feet, or apply with a cotton pad or cloth and rub in. Let dry before getting dressed. Follow with a natural deodorizing body powder, if desired.

This formula doubles as an astringent and mild antiseptic liquid cleanser for your hands, face, or entire body, for that matter (avoid the eyes, nose, and mouth). Use for impromptu cleansing when a bath or shower is not convenient. It also makes a good mosquito repellent.

Recipe excerpted from Stephanie Tourles' Essential Oils: A Beginner's Guide, *(©2018 by Stephanie Tourles). Used with permission from Storey Publishing.*

The Herbs of Ayurveda

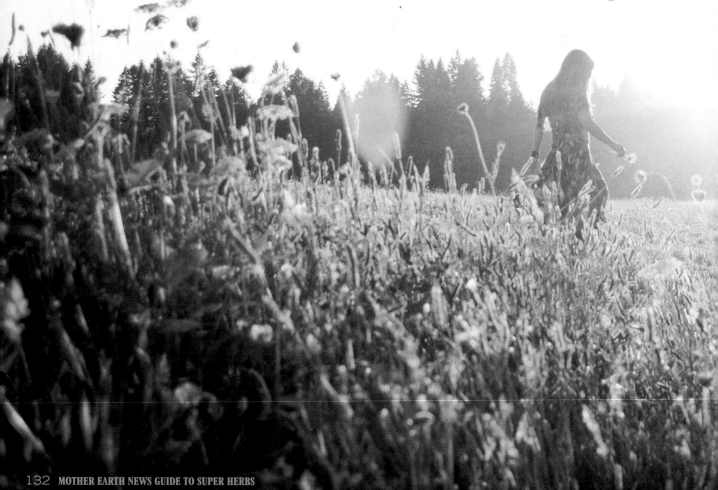

Ayurveda, the ancient Indian medicinal system, has been used for thousands of years to naturally support human health. Many of its main components focus on a healthful diet and the use of medicinal herbs. Read on to learn about some of the most popular Ayurvedic herbs, all of which have been used for centuries to promote holistic well-being.

By Jessica Kellner

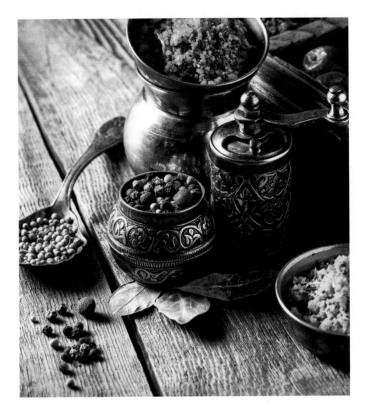

The ancient medicinal system known as Ayurveda looks at human health holistically, combining the physical with the mental and spiritual to create a sophisticated picture of health that encompasses all parts of a person. Some of the most critical components of Ayurveda include diet, meditation, and exercise—all of which are used to achieve balance in the body. Health is optimized when a person finds balance among the three doshas, or energies: vata, associated with respiration, circulation, elimination, movement, creativity, enthusiasm, and the nervous system; pitta, associated with transformations, including metabolism, digestion, vision, body temperature, intellect, courage, and cheerfulness; and kapha, associated with growth, lubrication, patience, fluid balance, compassion, and understanding.

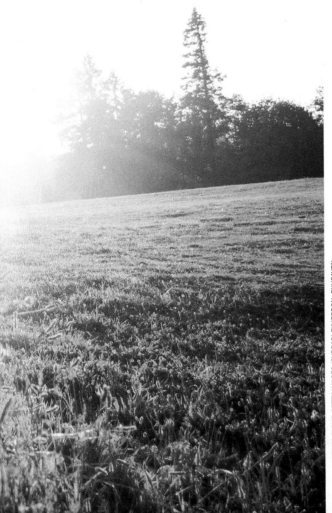

According to Ayurvedic theory, all people are made up of some combination of the three doshas. Most people have a dominant dosha, although some may be tri-dosha, or a fairly even combination of the three. To discover your own dosha, look for an entertaining online quiz such as the ones available from Nature's Formulary (Natures Formulary.com/test/Dosha-Test) or Maharishi Ayurveda (mapi.com/doshas/dosha-test/index.html). To seek medicinal advice based on Ayurvedic theory, consult a trained Ayurvedic specialist.

Used alongside diet, meditation, and exercise, the primary form of medicine in Ayurveda is herbs. Ayurvedic herbal medicines have been used to balance the doshas and promote health for thousands of years. Many people find these herbs' tonic effects beneficial—and they're especially relevant today as many are helpful for managing or reducing stress, regulating blood sugar and hormones, and aiding in proper digestion. It's a credit to the deeply holistic nature of Ayurveda that many of its primary objectives are equally or more important today as they may have been thousands of years ago. Read on to learn a bit about some of the premier herbal medicines recommended in Ayurveda. All of these herbs are generally safe and have been used for centuries—however, as always, exercise caution in the use of medicinal herbs, especially if you have chronic medical conditions, take prescription medications, or are pregnant or nursing.

Trikatu

Trikatu, translated to "three pungents," is a blend of black pepper, long pepper, and ginger. Considered medicinal and culinary, trikatu is said to be stimulative in nature; helpful for the liver, spleen, and pancreas; and increase bile production, aiding digestion. Because it contains piperine, it's frequently used in Ayurvedic formulations to help increase absorption of other medicines and is suggested for weight loss, to boost metabolism, and for diabetics. Trikatu is often used in concert with triphala; triphala is said to benefit the lower gastrointestinal (GI) tract, while trikatu is said to enhance digestion in the upper GI.

To Use: Combine powdered trikatu with honey, then take straight or add to green tea or tomato juice. You can also find capsules. A typical dosage is 125 to 500 mg twice daily, with food. Dosages beyond 1 gram daily may cause heartburn; do not exceed 1,000 mg a day.

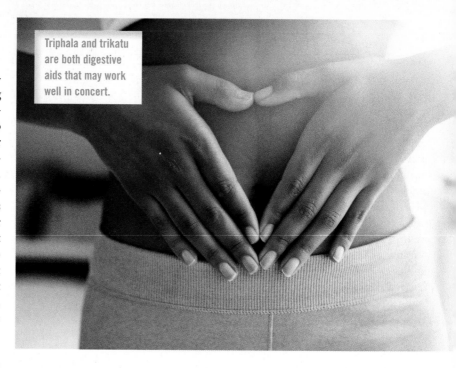

Triphala and trikatu are both digestive aids that may work well in concert.

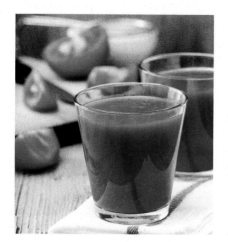

Triphala

Considered by many to be the most important treatment in Ayurvedic medicine, triphala is a combination of three fruits: Amalaki, also called Indian gooseberry, is full of vitamin C, supports healthy metabolism and digestion, and may help lower cholesterol; haritaki, known as the Tibetan "king of medicine," is anti-inflammatory and laxative, but can also relieve diarrhea; and bibhitaki, which is said to be a rejuvenator and detoxifier for the blood, muscles, and fatty tissues in the body. In Ayurveda, triphala is recommended for all dosha types and is considered something of a panacea. Triphala is most well-known for its abilities to improve digestion and elimination. According to Ayurvedic medicinal theory, all health begins with healthy digestion, and triphala is effective at treating various gastrointestinal disorders. Studies over the past two decades have shown triphala an effective free radical scavenger that's anti-inflammatory, antibacterial, antioxidant, adaptogenic, and anticancer. Although human studies in many of these areas are lacking, animal studies have found triphala capable of treating infections; managing gastrointestinal problems; controlling inflammation, cholesterol, and other markers associated with obesity; strengthening the immune system; and, in lab studies, treating cancer.

To Use: In Ayurveda, triphala is considered a useful herb for everyone. For maintenance, herbalist Karta Purkh Singh Khalsa recommends taking 2 grams daily; as a short-term laxative, take 6 grams daily.

Yoga, Breath, and Meditation: The Other Ayurvedic Keys to Health

Diet and herbs are key components of health in Ayurveda. Equally critical are physical movement and stress management using yoga, breath work (also known as pranayama), and meditation. One Ayurvedic doctor explains the relationship between yoga and Ayurveda like this, says Babeeta Chhabra, a yoga instructor associated with The Art of Living Retreat Center: "Ayurveda is the science and yoga is the practice of the science." Both yoga and Ayurveda advocate for the regular practice of pranayama and meditation.

The benefits of yoga, breath work, and meditation are all widely supported by modern research. Yoga is documented to improve body image; promote mindful eating, reducing emotional and distracted eating; support weight loss and weight maintenance; and enhance physical

Ashwagandha

Ashwagandha is an anti-inflammatory tonic used to help relieve stress and improve stamina. Animal studies have found ashwagandha to relax the central nervous system, making it useful for reducing stress and improving sleep quality. In one human study, eight weeks of use decreased stress, as well as food cravings and overall body weight. Ashwagandha also shows promise in fighting cancer. In lab tests, ashwagandha kills cancer cells and enhances immune cells; it may also enhance the effectiveness of radiation therapy. Human studies are needed. Ashwagandha has also been used to treat arthritis pain. In one study of 86 joint pain sufferers, treatment with ashwagandha and the Ayurvedic medicine Sidh Makardhwaj produced significant reductions in swollen joints and pain assessment scores. Finally, ashwagandha may aid in cognitive disorders, including Alzheimer's disease. In lab studies, researchers have found ashwagandha to inhibit formation of beta-amyloid plaques, neurotoxic plaques that accumulate in the brains of people with neurodegenerative disease. In studies on mice with Alzheimer's disease, treatment with ashwagandha significantly improved cognitive performance and reduced the presence of amyloid plaques.

To Use: Standardized extracts should include 2.5 to 5 percent anolides. Dosage varies — consult a medical professional, or choose a high-quality supplement and follow dosage instructions. Pregnant women shouldn't take ashwagandha.

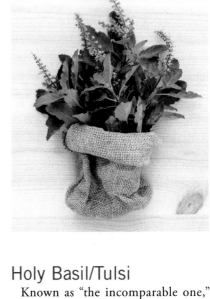

Holy Basil/Tulsi

Known as "the incomparable one," tulsi is considered sacred in the Hindu faith, and a large body of research supports the many traditional uses of the plant. Holy basil contains a variety of beneficial constituents, including ursolic acid and rosmarinic acid, both of which are also found in rosemary, as well as carotenoids, vitamin C, calcium, iron, zinc, and chlorophyll. Holy basil is known as a tonic herb used to help our bodies manage stress, and several studies back up this use. Holy basil is useful for promoting improved resilience to stress, recovery from chronic stress, and avoidance of chronic stress-induced physiological changes. Holy basil is highly antioxidant, cancer-protective, and cardioprotective — the herb has been shown to improve cardiovascular risk factors, including, in one animal study, reducing fasting blood glucose by 60 percent in the treatment group compared with 10 percent in a control group. Also useful for pain relief, holy basil has been shown to reduce arthritis swelling by up to 73 percent after 24 hours of treatment. It's recommended for skin health, helping restore skin's collagen structure and elasticity, as well as for wound healing. Holy basil is also recommended for diabetics, and several animal studies have found reduced fasting blood sugar, as well as glycemic-lowering properties.

To Use: Holy basil is often sold in tea form, and it can also be taken in capsules. A typical dose is 500 mg of leaf extract taken twice daily.

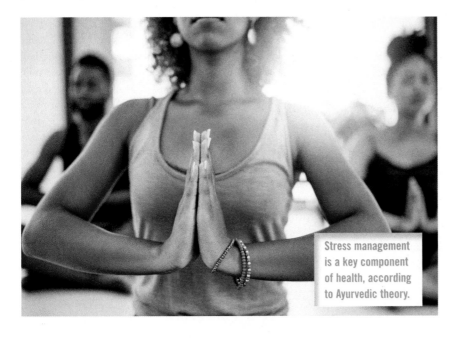

Stress management is a key component of health, according to Ayurvedic theory.

fitness, including muscle strength, endurance, flexibility, and cardiorespiratory fitness.

Breath work and meditation are well-documented to help mediate stress response, lower blood pressure, reduce chronic pain and headaches, improve sleep quality, and alleviate mild depression and anxiety.

To experience these benefits, enjoy a guided meditation program for free on YouTube, or try a paid program such as those offered from Headspace (Headspace.com). The best way to learn yoga is to attend a class with a qualified instructor who can guide you in proper form and technique. Many classes incorporate breathing exercises. Guided breathing exercises are also available online.

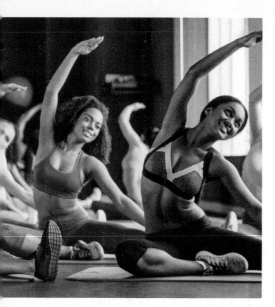

Shatavari

Shatavari is considered the premier women's herb in Ayurveda, and it's used to balance hormones, reduce symptoms of menopause and menstruation, increase lactation, reduce inflammation of sexual organs, and increase libido. Shatavari is a relative of the asparagus plant, and its name translates into either "having 100 roots" or "having 100 husbands," a name said to reference its benefits for all women. Although modern science has not investigated shatavari in depth, it's considered a useful tonic for women at all stages of life, and particularly useful for irritability surrounding menstruation. Shatavari's immune-modulating properties are its most well-researched — the herb has a measurable effect on the functioning of macrophages, important immune cells responsible for digesting potentially harmful organisms as well as cancer cells. Studies have also shown shatavari can enhance macrophages' ability to fight the fungus candida. It's also an effective digestive aid.

To Use: Shatavari is available as a powder or capsules. For PMS or menopausal symptoms, some experts recommend 500-mg capsules, up to 2 grams daily. To soothe digestion, try a teaspoon of powder mixed into milk after meals. Shatavari is also useful for those recovering from illness or surgery; however, always consult a physician before using it after surgery.

Bitter Melon

Eaten as a vegetable in Bangladesh and several other Asian countries, bitter melon is believed to be especially effective at warding off diabetes, obesity, and metabolic syndrome, all of which are becoming epidemic in both developed and developing nations. Containing numerous vitamins, minerals, antioxidants and phytochemicals, bitter melon is nutritious. In several studies, bitter melon extract has been shown to be beneficial in preventing body weight gain and visceral fat mass in rats fed high-fat diets. Research also shows bitter melon to be effective in the treatment of diabetes — both clinical and animal studies support its ability to lower blood glucose levels, improve insulin sensitivity, and improve glycogen synthesis in the liver. Bitter melon also demonstrates a protective effect against nonalcoholic fatty liver disease, mainly attributed to its antioxidant capacity to scavenge free radicals and reduce inflammation in the liver. The liver undergoes significant challenges during diet-induced obesity and diabetes, as excess fat intake overwhelms the organ's capacity to metabolize fats, causing oxidative stress. This is a component of the process leading to metabolic syndrome — the combination of symptoms that are a precursor for obesity, type 2 diabetes, and a number of other serious health concerns.

To Use: Bitter melon is often recommended as a food or juice, although many people find its taste unpleasant. The traditional preparation in Bangladesh is to stir-fry bitter melon with potatoes, garlic, chilies, and onion until some of the melon's strong odor is reduced. It's also available as a tincture or capsules, but many factors determine the appropriate dose. Don't attempt to use bitter melon to control diabetes without the advice of a trained medical professional. Bitter melon should not be used by pregnant or nursing women, or following surgery.

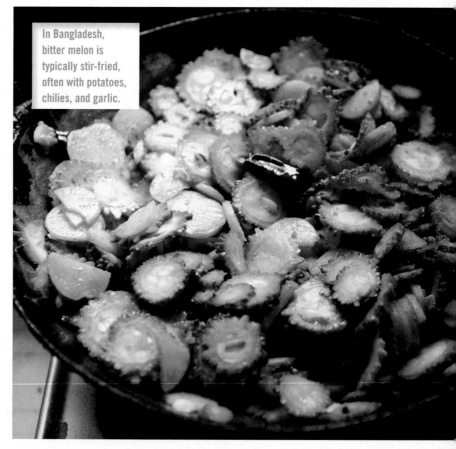

In Bangladesh, bitter melon is typically stir-fried, often with potatoes, chilies, and garlic.

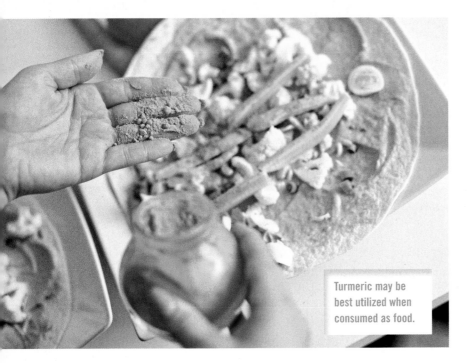

Turmeric may be best utilized when consumed as food.

Turmeric

An herb whose medicinal benefits have become increasingly famed in recent years, turmeric has long been prized as a beneficial food and spice in Indian and other Asian cultures. Turmeric is a powerful antioxidant, which benefits nearly all bodily systems. It's said to improve digestion; assist in the proper functioning of cells; support the brain and nervous system; maintain joint mobility; support healthy blood sugar levels and proper liver function; nourish the circulatory system; and boost immunity. Turmeric is highly anti-inflammatory, which is why it's often recommended for joint conditions, including arthritis. Studies suggest turmeric may help prevent atherosclerosis, the buildup of plaque that can block arteries, leading to heart attack or stroke. Preliminary research in test tube and animal studies suggests curcumin, a component of turmeric, may help prevent several types of cancers, including those of the prostate, breast, skin, and colon. Yet some researchers say turmeric has been overhyped in recent years; in a review of the medicinal chemistry of curcumin published in the *Journal of Medicinal Chemistry*, researchers found no double-blind, placebo-controlled studies (the gold standard for scientists) that supported the herb's many health claims. One reason they believe curcumin may not live up to its hype is its low bioavailability—on its own, the body has difficulty with uptake of curcumin. This has long been known, however, which is why it's often recommended to consume turmeric along with black pepper and fat, both of which enhance its bioavailability. Certainly, consuming turmeric as food—such as in curries or golden milk—is beneficial, despite questions about its efficacy when used as a supplement.

To Use: If possible, consume turmeric as a regular part of the diet in curries, golden milk, stews, soups, stir-fries, or even atop oatmeal or mixed into pancake batter. If you choose supplements, choose those in which whole turmeric is combined with piperine, a component of black pepper that helps increase curcumin's absorption. Piperine can slow the elimination of some prescription drugs from the bloodstream, so consult a physician before combining a piperine-containing supplement with prescription medication. Pregnant women should seek a doctor's approval before using turmeric supplements. Turmeric may also interfere with some chemotherapy drugs used to treat breast cancer.

Brahmi

Brahmi (*Bacopa monnieri*), also known as bacopa (and often confused with gotu kola, a similar herb also called brahmi in northern India), is prized for its cognitive benefits; is said to improve mental performance and memory; can stimulate the cerebrovascular system; and may relax the nervous system, making it useful to calm anxiety and panic attacks. In one study, 76 adults age 40 to 65 saw a significant improvement in the retention of new information after taking brahmi. In several small studies on children, brahmi has been found to improve immediate memory, reaction time, logical memory, and concentration. Studies also suggest brahmi may be useful in the prevention of oxidative stress, often linked with neurodegenerative disease. Because of its effects on the nervous system, brahmi is used to relieve stress and stress-induced insomnia. Recent research also suggests brahmi may be useful in treating ADHD. In one clinical trial, ADHD-diagnosed children who took brahmi for 12 weeks saw significant improvements on all tested parameters, including mental control, logical memory, word recall, and more.

To Use: To relieve stress/anxiety, take 50 to 100 mg three times a day (effects take two to three months). Studies on mental function have used 300 mg a day. Brahmi is fat-soluble and can upset stomachs, so take it with fat-containing food. Consult a medical professional before using it in children. 🌳

Jessica Kellner was the editor in chief of *Mother Earth Living* magazine.

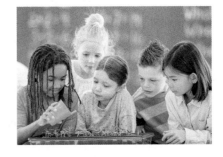

A CLOSER LOOK AT MULTIVITAMINS

Is taking multivitamins healthful, wishful thinking, or harmful?

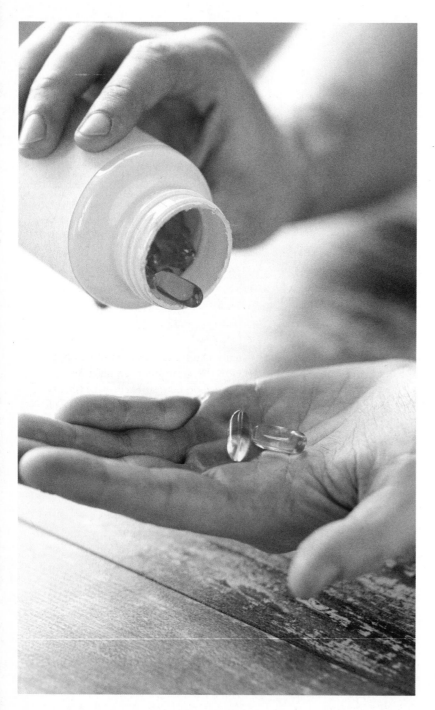

By Linda B. White

When I was a child, I remember washing down a multivitamin and mineral (MVM) supplement with my orange juice each morning. That red pill fell into the same category as brushing my teeth, eating my vegetables, and spending time outdoors—all daily activities somehow linked to health.

Apparently, I wasn't alone. Supplement use is common in the U.S.: One-third of Americans take a daily MVM supplement, according to a 2011 study. The question is, why? Most people probably expect a daily multivitamin will make them feel better and prevent common illnesses, but evidence behind these claims is uncertain—does taking a daily multivitamin help boost resistance to disease, or does it do more harm than good?

Why Do We Take Multivitamins?

"Historically, vitamin and mineral supplements were used to prevent diseases caused by deficiency," says Ann Diker, chair of the Health Professions Department at Metropolitan State University of Denver. Yet vitamin and mineral deficiencies aren't common in the U.S. Today, Americans consume many processed foods, and much of it is fortified with vitamins and minerals—a report from the Centers for Disease Control and Prevention states that a fortification of foods with folate (a B vitamin) has reduced deficiency to less than 1 percent, and deficiency of vitamins A and E are also uncommon.

There are exceptions: For example, those living in poverty face food insecurity (unreliable access to high-quality food). Elderly people are generally more at risk for deficiency. Vegans often need to supplement with vitamin B12, Diker notes. Kids, menstruating women, and pregnant women are more at risk for iron deficiency. Yet overall, the majority of us aren't deficient in major nutrients. And if we are, it is a single deficiency.

So what's our motivation for paying good money for MVMs? "Busy people don't take the time to plan a diet that would supply all their vitamins and minerals," Diker says. "So they take a MVM as a form of insurance." What's not clear is whether that insurance policy pays off.

Multivitamin Studies

A common expectation is that MVMs will prevent illnesses. However, most studies have not shown significant benefits in American adults. For example, in 2009 data from the Women's Health Initiative (or WHI, a long-term national health study of postmenopausal women) judged that routine use of MVMs had no significant impact on longevity, the development of cardiovascular disease or several common cancers.

Multivitamins also appear not to benefit cognitive or cardiovascular health. Two studies published in the *Annals of Internal Medicine* in 2013 found that a multivitamin failed to improve cognitive function in older men and did not reduce cardiovascular events in patients after a recent myocardial infarction.

Yet multivitamins may help protect older people against cancer death. A 2013 study of postmenopausal women (ages 50 to 79) enrolled in the WHI found that, among women who had been diagnosed with invasive breast cancer taking MVMs around the time of diagnosis, the risk of death from breast cancer was 30 percent lower relative to women not taking MVMs.

Sylvia Wassertheil-Smoller, a doctor at Albert Einstein College of Medicine in Bronx, New York, was the principal investigator in both WHI studies. Her view is that MVMs don't seem to benefit healthy people eating proper diets. However, due to biological and socioeconomic changes associated with aging, older adults are more at risk for inadequate nutrition. "Although the supplements didn't prevent cancer, they may have helped these older women

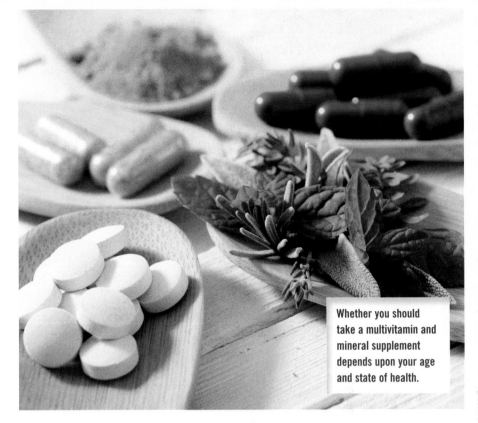

Whether you should take a multivitamin and mineral supplement depends upon your age and state of health.

withstand the assault of cancer once it took hold," Wassertheil-Smoller says.

A 2012 study followed 14,000 male physicians aged 50 and older for more than a decade and found that a daily multivitamin (Centrum Silver) reduced the number of new cases of cancer by 8 percent, but did not impact the number of deaths.

When it comes to nutrients, more is not better. While deficiency can lead to ill health, excessive intake of some vitamins and minerals can be toxic—particularly fat-soluble vitamins such as vitamins A, E, and K, which accumulate in the body. The Iowa Women's Health Study evaluated the impact of a number of vitamin and mineral supplements on the risk of cancer, cardiovascular disease, and death in older women over an 18-year period. A number of individual supplements such as iron and particularly copper were associated with an increased risk of death. Fortunately, MVMs were associated with a smaller risk. Lead researcher Jaakko Mursua, doctor at the Institute of Public Health and Clinical Nutrition, University of Eastern Finland, Kuopio, notes that most similar studies found no evidence for harm. In Wassertheil-Smoller's studies, MVMs appear to be safe.

Should You Take a Multivitamin?

So should you take MVMs? The answer depends upon your age and state of health. "Children generally don't need to take vitamin and mineral supplements," says Mary Kohn, assistant professor of pediatrics at the University of Colorado.

"Picky eaters may benefit from a daily children's multivitamin to provide the vitamins they need and to avoid food battles. Exclusively breast-fed babies should receive 400 IU of vitamin D from age 2 months until they're taking solid foods."

All pregnant and breast-feeding women (and those planning pregnancies) should take prenatal vitamin supplements that contain folic acid, crucial for proper nervous system development, says Kate Koschoreck, nurse-midwife at the University of Colorado. Wassertheil-Smoller's attitude for adults older than 50 is, "These multivitamins do no harm and may do good if a women develops breast cancer. So why not take them?"

Healthy, well-nourished adolescents and adults don't usually need MVMs. Most health professionals say whole foods trump supplements every time

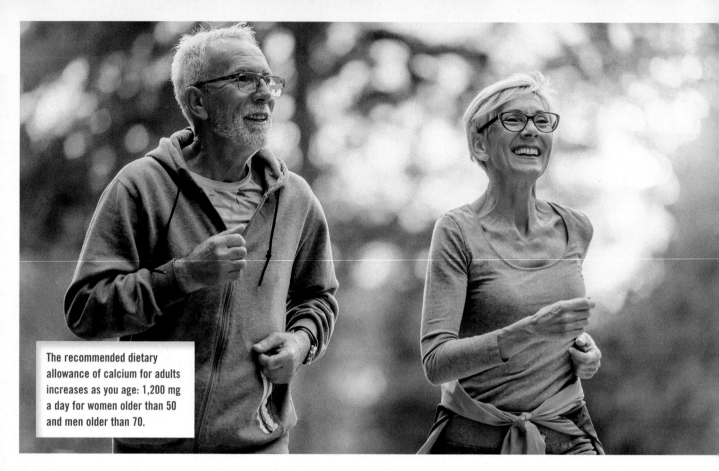

The recommended dietary allowance of calcium for adults increases as you age: 1,200 mg a day for women older than 50 and men older than 70.

because food — particularly plant food — is chemically complex, containing much more than the vitamins and minerals you get in a pill. If you have any doubts, consult your doctor. Tests can determine whether you are deficient in a particular vitamin or mineral.

Other Dietary Supplements

This article only addresses multivitamin and mineral formulas. A host of other supplements exist: single vitamins and minerals, amino acids, essential fatty acids, hormones, herbal extracts, and more. These supplements may be appropriate to help treat or prevent certain illnesses or conditions. Consult your physician.

5 Super Supplements

So should I take supplements, and if so what should I take? It's not an easy question to answer. While we all want to make sure we are protecting our (and our family's) health by working toward achieving ideal nutrition, we also don't want to spend hundreds of dollars and pop dozens of pills. The fact is that if you regularly eat high-quality whole

foods, your gastrointestinal tract functions well, and you're usually healthy, then you probably don't need many dietary supplements.

However, some nutrients are vital or highly beneficial, and our diets simply may not be providing enough of them. Even if we strive to live a healthy lifestyle, many of us fall outside the area of "ideal" health and nutrition. Sometimes we lack the time, money, or inclination to prepare perfectly wholesome meals every day. With age and illness, intestines may not efficiently absorb nutrients, and acute and chronic diseases increase demands for certain nutrients. To be sure, supplement needs vary by individual, but these five are the most often-recommended dietary supplements. If you have questions, always check with your doctor.

1. Calcium

Bones, nerves, muscles, hormones, and enzymes need calcium. Blood levels are maintained at a fairly even keel, and if they drop, calcium is removed from bone. It's crucial that we don't run a long-term deficit.

Dosage: The recommended dietary

allowance (RDA) for adults is 1,000 mg a day. The intake increases to 1,200 mg a day for women older than 50 and men older than 70.

Other sources: If we eat well, we should be able to satisfy the requirements from food. Most experts say the best way to get calcium is from cruciferous vegetables (especially dark-green leafy vegetables), dairy products, sardines, peanuts, sesame seeds, sunflower seeds, dried beans, figs, and seaweed.

Deficiency: Many people, particularly those older than 70, fall short of recommended calcium intake without supplements. For instance, women 50 to 70 typically get about 780 mg of calcium from food. Long-term deficiency increases risk for osteoporosis.

Pros & cons: For decades, doctors routinely recommended calcium supplements. The side effects seemed relatively minor — mainly constipation and bloating. On the other hand, the risk of a devastating, osteoporosis-related bone fracture declined 12 percent with calcium plus vitamin D supplementation. Then, in 2010, two reports linked calcium supplementation with a 24 to 31 percent increased risk of heart

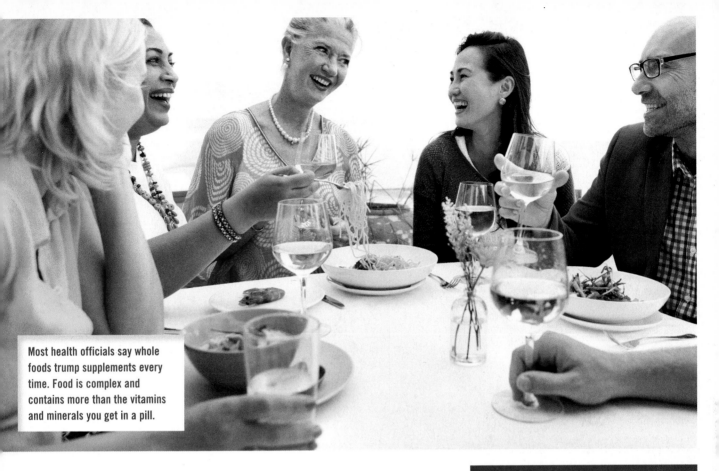

Most health officials say whole foods trump supplements every time. Food is complex and contains more than the vitamins and minerals you get in a pill.

attacks. Other research has not shown cardiovascular risks.

Always try to obtain your calcium from food, says Douglas C. Bauer, a doctor and professor of medicine, epidemiology and biostatistics at the University of California, San Francisco. For those unable to do so, Bauer recommends one of two types of calcium supplements: calcium carbonate and calcium citrate.

Less-expensive calcium carbonate contains a higher percentage of calcium (40 percent), but it's more likely to cause constipation and bloating. Adequate absorption requires stomach acid, which declines with age. If you're older than 60 or take an antacid, use calcium citrate. A typical calcium citrate dosage is one 1,000-mg tablet, two to three times a day, or 420 to 630 mg of calcium. Don't exceed 2,500 mg of calcium in food and supplements a day.

2. Magnesium

Like calcium, magnesium is a major mineral in the body that contributes to bone structure. It's also required for many chemical reactions; nerve and muscle function; protein synthesis; energy production; blood pressure and heart rate regulation; and blood sugar control.

Dosage: The RDA varies depending on age and gender. For men 19 to 30, the RDA is 400 mg, thereafter rising to 420 mg. The RDA for women 19 to 30 is 310 mg; 320 mg for those nursing a baby or older than 31; and 360 mg during pregnancy.

Other sources: Particularly good food sources are green leafy vegetables, legumes, whole grains, avocados, seeds, and nuts.

Deficiency: National health surveys show that nearly half of kids and adults fail to consume adequate amounts of dietary magnesium: Among teens 14 to 18, and adults older than 70, more than two-thirds don't get enough magnesium.

People at higher risk for magnesium deficiency include those with kidney disease, intestinal disorders (for example, celiac disease and Crohn's disease), type 2 diabetes, alcohol dependence, and the elderly. Used long-term, some diuretics and proton pump inhibitors (drugs such as Nexium and Prevacid) can cause magnesium

"Even if we strive to live a healthy lifestyle, many of us fall outside the area of 'ideal' health and nutrition."

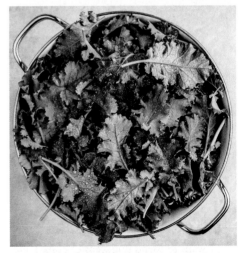

Many experts agree that dark-green leafy vegetables are a great source of calcium and magnesium.

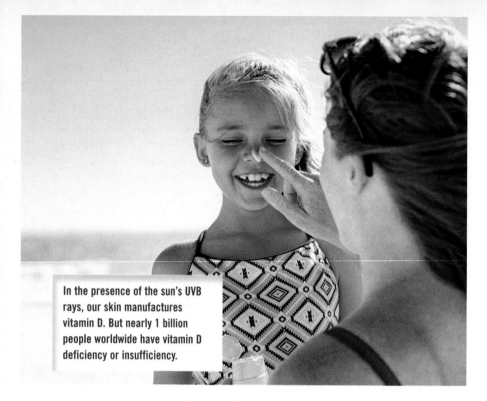

In the presence of the sun's UVB rays, our skin manufactures vitamin D. But nearly 1 billion people worldwide have vitamin D deficiency or insufficiency.

the process; darker-skinned people require more UVB exposure to generate vitamin D; vitamin D production becomes less efficient as we age; and winter sunlight in much of the northern U.S. is too weak to stimulate the process.

Only a few foods contain much vitamin D: oily fish, eggs (from vitamin D-fed hens), sun-exposed mushrooms, and fortified products including dairy, soy milk, orange juice, and cereals.

Deficiency: About 1 billion people worldwide have vitamin D deficiency (blood levels less than 20 ng/mL) or insufficiency (21 to 29 ng/mL), says Michael F. Holick, a doctor, researcher, and professor of medicine at Boston University School of Medicine. Vitamin D deficiency causes skeletal deformities in children, and osteomalacia (a painful softening of the bones) and osteoporosis in adults. Deficiency can lead to falls and bone fractures, and has been linked to a higher risk of cardiovascular disease; some cancers; respiratory infections; asthma; and autoimmune disorders such as multiple sclerosis, depression, diabetes, reduced fertility, and Alzheimer's-type dementia.

Groups at risk for insufficiency include breast-fed infants; older adults; people who are obese; people with scant exposure to the sun; people with liver or kidney disease; and those with intestinal diseases or surgeries that limit fat absorption. Pregnant women require adequate vitamin D to ensure normal fetal bone development.

Pros & cons: Because we don't get much vitamin D from food (about 200 IU a day), many health authorities recommend supplements, starting in infancy. The Endocrine Society, an international organization dedicated to research and education about hormones, recommends daily supplementation as follows to prevent deficiency:

- Infants 0 to 12 months: 400 to 1,000 IU; don't exceed 2,000 IU
- Children and adolescents between 1 and 18: 600 to 1,000 IU; don't exceed 4,000 IU

deficiency. Most people — unless extremely malnourished or ill — don't develop signs of severe magnesium deficiency. Early signs include reduced appetite, nausea, vomiting, fatigue, and weakness. Suboptimal magnesium intake can, over time, increase risk of high blood pressure, cardiovascular disease, stroke, type 2 diabetes, osteoporosis, and migraines.

Pros & cons: When you shop for supplements, you'll see that magnesium is always bound to another chemical. Magnesium bound to aspartate, citrate, lactate, and chloride forms is better absorbed and more bioavailable than magnesium oxide and magnesium sulfate. Magnesium supplements can correct low blood levels of magnesium (a condition detected by a blood test). Studies show that higher intakes of magnesium from food and supplements combined reduced the risk of developing type 2 diabetes. Although results are mixed, some studies show that magnesium supplements improve insulin sensitivity in people who already have type 2 diabetes. Supplements also show promise for people with migraines, premenstrual syndrome (PMS), high cholesterol, and coronary artery disease.

Your dosage should depend upon how much you're getting from food, your age, sex, the condition you're trying to treat, and whether or not you're deficient. As always, it's better not to exceed the RDA.

While the kidneys do a good job of eliminating excess, high intake from supplements can trigger diarrhea, intestinal cramping, and nausea. (Some commercial laxatives are magnesium-based.) The good news is that if you take calcium supplements, magnesium counteracts their constipating effect.

3. Vitamin D

Vitamin D promotes calcium absorption from the intestines. Its multiple functions include bone mineralization, cell growth, and reduction of inflammation. It's also involved in the function of nerves, muscles, and the immune system.

Dosage: The RDA is 400 IU for infants younger than a year, 600 IU for children and adults, and 800 IU for people older than 70.

Other sources: In the presence of the sun's UVB rays, our skin manufactures vitamin D. A few facts to keep in mind: Sunscreen can interfere with

GETTY IMAGES/RIDOFRANZ

• Adults older than 18: 1,500 to 2,000 IU; don't exceed 10,000 IU

If you're in one of the groups at risk for deficiency, ask your doctor for a blood test for 25-hydroxyvitamin D to better determine your optimal supplement dose. Excessive vitamin D can elevate blood levels of calcium, leading to damage to kidneys, heart, and blood vessels. Sun exposure does not lead to vitamin D overdose.

4. Fish Oil

Fatty fish are rich in the omega-3 fatty acids docosapentaenoic acid, eicosapentaenoic acid (EPA), and docosahexaenoic acid (DHA)—critical to fetal development and health throughout life, says Robert C. Block, a doctor at the University of Rochester School of Medicine and Dentistry in Rochester, New York. They become incorporated into many parts of the body (notably cell membranes), and have anti-inflammatory effects.

Dosage: Many health experts recommend consuming fatty fish once or twice a week, or taking supplements. The government doesn't set RDAs for fatty acids, but typical fish oil doses in studies range from 1 to 4 grams a day. Because of the importance of EPA and DHA during

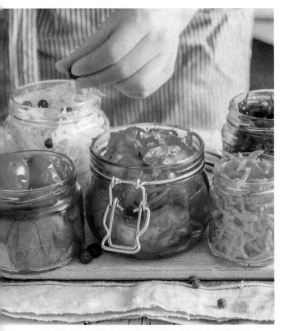

ermented foods naturally contain beneficial microbes, and is a great way to get good bacteria into your gut.

fetal and infant development, adequate intake is particularly important for pregnant and nursing women.

Other sources: Fish is the best dietary source for preformed EPA and DHA. However, algal sources are becoming increasingly available.

Deficiency: Fatty acids come in two main varieties: omega-3 and omega-6. Modern diets often contain too little of the former and too much of the latter. Signs of essential fatty acid deficiency include poor growth and development in infants and children, dry scaly rash, increased susceptibility to infection, and poor wound healing. Low levels of EPA and DHA are associated with inflammatory conditions, cardiovascular disease, reduced cognitive function, and some psychological disorders (attention deficit hyperactivity disorder, depression, and bipolar disorder).

Pros & cons: Getting adequate fatty acids is crucial. Eating fatty fish seems to reduce the risk of developing heart disease. (However, recent studies show fish oil supplementation offers no reduction in death, heart attack, or stroke in people at risk for cardiovascular disease.) In people who already have heart disease, supplements reduce deaths, but don't seem to protect against so-called "cardiovascular events" (heart attacks and strokes).

Fatty acid intake affects inflammation levels and brain health. Preliminary research suggests fish and fish oil supplements decrease breast cancer risk. The brain depends upon adequate amounts of omega-3 fatty acids, especially DHA. Diets high in these oils protect against age-related cognitive decline and Alzheimer's disease. Preliminary evidence of benefits also exist (as adjuncts to conventional treatment) of dietary fish and fish oil supplements in attention deficit hyperactivity disorder, asthma, and age-related macular degeneration. In terms of side effects, fish oil supplements may cause fishy-tasting burps, heartburn, and nausea, but no major health risks.

5. Probiotics

Probiotics are live microorganisms (bacteria and yeast) similar to those already residing in our intestinal tract. Our normal "gut flora" benefit us by outcompeting disease-causing microbes, enhancing immune function, maintaining mucous membrane health, optimizing digestion, and manufacturing vitamins.

Dosage: There is no RDA; dosage is based on the number of colony forming units (CFUs) per capsule and range from 1 to 10 billion CFUs daily, divided.

Other sources: Fermented foods (yogurt, kefir, cultured buttermilk, unpasteurized sauerkraut, kimchi, miso, natto, tempeh) naturally contain beneficial microbes.

Deficiency: While it's impossible to be "deficient" in probiotics, it's common to have an ecologic disturbance in gut flora. Scientists link imbalances to diarrhea, asthma, irritable bowel syndrome, type 1 and 2 diabetes, obesity, and possibly cardiovascular disease.

Pros & cons: Preliminary research usually focuses on specific strains of bacteria (*Lactobacillus* or *Bifidobacteria*) and yeast (*Saccharomyces boulardii*). Positive studies exist for viral diarrhea in children (specifically rotavirus); diarrhea associated with antibiotics and chemotherapy; diarrhea caused by Clostridium difficile; traveler's diarrhea; eczema; bacterial vaginosis; infantile colic; and inflammatory bowel disease and irritable bowel syndrome. Prophylactic use may reduce the severity and frequency of respiratory infections. Probiotics appear to be safe when taken within dosage guidelines. If you have a colicky baby and want to try probiotics, talk to your pediatrician.

Linda B. White, M.D. works as a lecturer and freelance writer. Her most recent books are *Health Now* and *500 Time-Tested Home Remedies and the Science Behind Them*, coauthored with Barbara Seeber and Barbara Brownell Grogan (available at www. MotherEarthNews.com/Store).

"Before healing others,
heal yourself."
—Gambian proverb

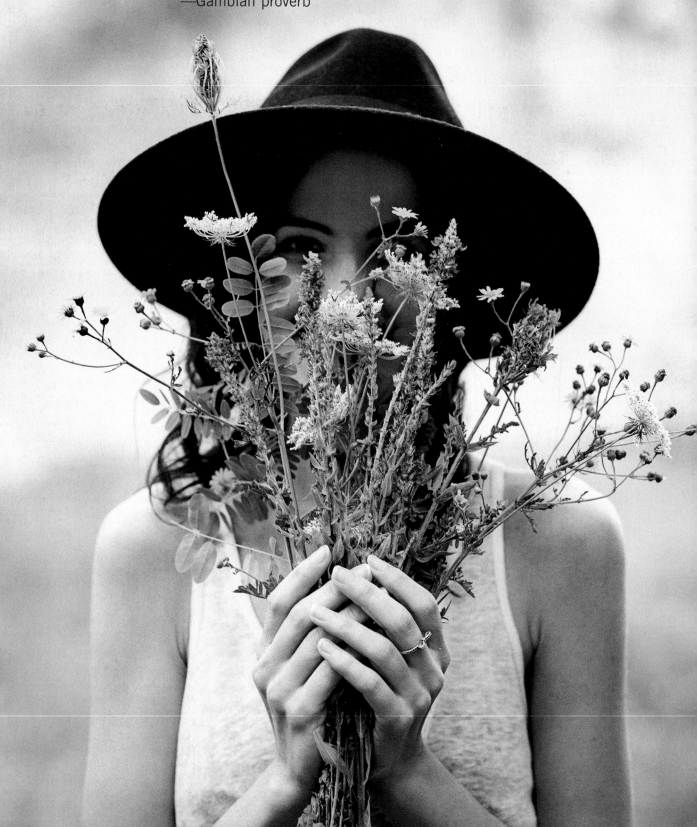